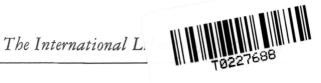
THE GROUP APPROACH TO
LEADERSHIP-TESTING

Founded by C. K. Ogden

The International Library of Psychology

SOCIAL PSYCHOLOGY
In 7 Volumes

I	Personal Aggressiveness and War	*Durbin et al*
II	The Psychology of Politics	*Eysenck*
III	Dynamic Social Research	*Hader et al*
IV	The Group Approach to Leadership-Testing	*Harris*
V	Co-operation, Tolerance, and Prejudice	*Lowy*
VI	Man and His Fellowmen	*Lowy*
VII	The Symbolic Process and its Integration in Children	*Markey*

THE GROUP APPROACH TO
LEADERSHIP-TESTING

HENRY HARRIS

Foreword by General Sir Ronald Adam

Preface by Brigadier A Torrie

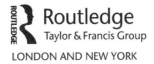

Routledge
Taylor & Francis Group

LONDON AND NEW YORK

First published in 1939
by Routledge
2 Park Square, Milton Park, Abingdon, Oxfordshire OX14 4RN
711 Third Avenue, New York, NY 10017

First issued in paperback 2014

Routledge is an imprint of the Taylor and Francis Group, an informa business

British Library Cataloguing in Publication Data
A CIP catalogue record for this book
is available from the British Library

The Group Approach to Leadership-Testing
ISBN 0415-21119-0
Social Psychology: 7 Volumes
ISBN 0415-21134-4
The International Library of Psychology: 204 Volumes
ISBN 0415-19132-7

ISBN 13: 978-1-138-87575-3 (pbk)
ISBN 13: 978-0-415-21119-2 (hbk)

CONTENTS

PAGE

Foreword by General Sir Ronald Adam, Bt.,
G.C.B., D.S.O., O.B.E.   vii

Preface by Brigadier A. Torrie   .   .   .   ix

PART I: THEORIES

CHAP.

I Introduction   1

II The Field or Group Approach in Psychology   .   5

III The Group   10

IV The Leader   19

V The Leaderless Group or Stress Group Task   .   26

PART II: TECHNIQUES

PRELIMINARY PROCEDURES

VI General Plan of 3-Phase WOSB Testing   .   .   39

VII The Reception of Candidates   49

VIII Psychological Screening by Written Tests: The
Projection Battery: The Personality Pointer   .   52

PHASE 1: OBSERVERS FUNCTION AS A TEAM

IX Phase 1: Getting the General Pattern of the
Candidates Group-effectiveness: The Basic
Series   74

X How to Conduct, Interpret, Evaluate and Report
the Leaderless Group   85

XI The Query Conference or First Interphase Screen   101

PHASE 2: THE OBSERVER TEAM SPLITS

XII Phase 2: Differentiating Group-effectiveness into
its Component Roles: the PSO Battery and
Interviews   109

XIII Interpersonal Relationships and the Human
Problems Session   123

XIV The Projective Psychiatric Interview   .   .   .   148

XV The Interim Grading Slip or Second Interphase
Screen   198

PHASE 3: THE OBSERVER TEAM RE-FORMS

CHAP.   PAGE
XVI Phase 3: Resolution of Discrepancies and Con-
     firmation: The Final Exercise   .   .   .   200
XVII A Sociometric Check-up: The Test of Objective
     Judgement   202

FINAL AND GENERAL PROCEDURES
XVIII The Final Board as the Last Screen .   .   .   210
  XIX The Functions of the Psychological Department .   227
  XX The Validation of Boards, Observers and Selection
      Procedures. By Major Gavin Reeve, M.Sc. .   234

PART III: TRENDS AND IMPLICATIONS

XXI   Leadership-testing in Other than Military
      Fields   251
XXII Participation in Collective Leadership as a True
      Social Incentive   256
XXIII A Note of Coordination   267
      Bibliographic Note   271
      Appendices:
          A—A Spectrum Rating of Officer Personality .   273
          B—A Self-briefing Proforma for the Socio-
             metric Test   275
          C—The Profile Proforma for the Final Board .   277
          D—The Interim Grading Slip   .   .   .   279
          E—A Short Interests Questionnaire   .   .   280
      Name Index   283
      Subject Index   284

FOREWORD

By GENERAL SIR RONALD ADAM, Bt.,
G.C.B., D.S.O., O.B.E.

Adjutant-General of the Forces 1941–46
Chairman of the British Council

This book, as the author states, is not an official account of Officer Selection in the Army. An official book will be published later, but it is important that those who took part in this experiment should record their impressions, and the author has had opportunities of seeing officer selection in action at first hand.

The Army, during the early days of the war, carried out its selection of candidates for training as officers by interview boards. It was clear that these were not being successful. The failure rate at OCTUS was high, and I know one course at an OCTU when 50 per cent of the course failed to pass out. This was a waste of time and had unfortunate effects even on good candidates, for the knowledge of a high failure rate did not give confidence to those attending.

The interview had a deterrrent effect on potential officers too. The average candidate did not feel that he was being given a fair chance, and there was a completely mistaken impression that the questions asked favoured the public school boy at the expense of those not so educated.

The decision to change the old methods was taken after a trial board, when groups of presidents interviewed candidates and recorded their opinions separately. This showed so marked a difference of the opinions expressed on the same candidate that a new method had to be found.

Early experiments were based on the tests which the German Army had employed from 1923 onwards, apparently to their satisfaction, but these were not a success.

The experimental board, which tested its methods by judging the officers attending a Company Commanders School, produced a system that showed promising results and these were continually improved until the system described by the author evolved.

The first board set up under the new system proved that the candidate considered that it was a great improvement on the old interview. In the Command in which it worked the number of volunteers for commissions went up by 25 per cent. It is to be remembered that no one could be forced to take a commission.

Great efforts were made to validate results, but the Army was working against time in producing the continual stream of officers required by units, and validation could not be complete. To my mind, the best validation was that the candidates going before the boards were satisfied that they had been given a fair chance to show their mettle and there was no discrimination or favouritism.

The officer in a modern army is a trainer of men as well as a leader. A certain standard of education is essential, if he is to learn his job and train his men. Had Great Britain had a higher school-leaving age and proper Adult Education, we should not have been faced, as we were towards the end of the war, with a shortage of officers. I believe that a scientific validation of the methods used in officer selection will be published next year, but I congratulate the author on having gone ahead in the production of this book. At a time when the question of the methods of choosing students for Universities is under examination, the possibility of selection methods used by the War Office Selection Boards, adopted by the French and Belgian Armies, and later by the Civil Service Selection Board, should be considered.

25th October, 1948

PREFACE

By BRIGADIER A. TORRIE

Formerly Director of Army Psychiatry

This book meets a need expressed during the debate in the House of Lords in May 1948 on the quality of candidates for the senior Civil Service. One of the noble Lords complained of lack of information about the method and rationale of scientific selection for leadership devised and developed in the Army Psychiatric Service and adopted by the Civil Service Selection Board.

The author is a medical psychologist with an unusually wide general experience of investigation in the field of human personality and with a considerable range of special experience in selection: with NCOs and "Other Ranks", potential officers and with officers chosen for special jobs i.e. for the Parachute and Glider Regiments, as Personnel Selection Officers, ex-prisoner-of-war officers for re-assignment to special posts, ATS officers etc. His skill and understanding have led to a consistent and far greater measured efficiency and ability to predict success in leadership roles than that of a selection board acting without his assistance. Careful research and validation has shown this.

To give the best results, it is essential that selection boards should have the assistance of a medical psychologist who has been trained to assess personality in depth. The analogy of building a house might illustrate the point. The military members of a board may be likened to the prospective owners. They know their needs and can represent them to the technicians. The architect and draughtsman deal with design and measurement and quantities of materials required etc. They are the homologues of the non-medical psychologists who measure intelligence, aptitudes and abilities. Yet no one would build a house on sand. The surveyor with his knowledge of geology has to assess the nature of the sub-soil on which the building has to be erected in order to ascertain its capacity to withstand the stresses it will be submitted to. In the same way the medical psychologist with his experience in analysing the springs of human personality is

necessary for the assessment of the capacity to withstand the
stresses and strains of the leadership role.   He can ascertain
the mechanisms of adaptability to environmental influences
present in spite of superficial evidences of eccentricity.

Researches have demonstrated that the medical psychologist
passes good men otherwise rejected by the non-technical members
of the board.   This may account for the high failure rate and
complaints in selection boards lacking those members who
planned and developed the procedure.   Without technical
members the procedure is parallel to the use of a stethoscope by
a layman who hears sounds but cannot interpret their meaning.

Validation has clearly shown the value of WOSB as
originally constituted with a full team including a medical
psychologist and a psychological officer.   The chapter on validation by Major Reeve indicates the degree of precision with
which these methods can be used and how selection boards may
be helped to keep on increasing their efficiency.

Our future prosperity we are told depends on an increase in
industrial productivity.   I hope that this book will help industry
to select the kind of leader who will achieve results by a knowledge and use of the human factor which the author has brought
to modern methods of selection.

11*th November* 1948

PART I: THEORIES

CHAPTER I

INTRODUCTION

Can leaders be picked and if so, how? The implications of any technique—sufficiently scientific and reliable—for selecting the potential leaders in a community are obviously tremendous. The truest wealth of a nation lies in its brains, character and leadership; and the germinating point of its culture resides in such of its brains and leadership as it can transmute from potentiality into realisation. Leadership and intelligence—like other human functions—are inherited only as potentialities; they must be made as well as born; they must be discovered, cherished, trained and given scope.

Any technique for discovering potential leadership while still trainable is of special import to Britain today, when with her 40 millions she must compete as well as co-operate (full co-operation is the hope of the future) with USA and USSR with 3 to 5 times her population. When she must produce so much to pay for her war and to maintain her standards with a diminished empire that she must perforce use *all* her leadership and brains and not merely some of it. When the way in which she uses her potential leadership will be not only a test of her democracy and a possible example and lead to the world but a very condition of her survival as a culture. For Britain there would seem to be no choice between quality or quantity, no dilemma: it *must* be quality if she is to survive significantly.

The British Army developed the basis of such a technique during 1942–1945 and in so doing made what one considers to be the major psychological contribution of the war. The techniques of psychological therapy, propaganda, education etc used, were so far as one knows derivative from the past: techniques and principles of leadership-testing however have had to be thrashed out from their very beginning. Developed in crisis—soon after Dunkirk—their prime purpose was to select junior leaders in a military field. It will be submitted here that with suitable modifications they can be used to select leaders in any field: derivative techniques are, or have been, used in the Civil Service, the National Fire Service, the Palestine Police, the India Office, the RAF, etc.

These psychological techniques resulted from the collective effort of many minds co-operating in War Office Selection Boards (popularly known as "Wosbies" from their initials WOSB) since 1942. First experiments were made with the help of a number of psychiatrists and psychologists i.e. Sutherland, Bion, Wittkower, Rodger, Trist etc. As the number of WOSBs grew, an experimental attitude was encouraged; the framework of testing was elastic, and principles and techniques were continuously being experimented with: there was in some Boards an atmosphere of fermenting creativity; as at the Research and Training Centre where the results of all experiments were integrated, evaluated and validated.

The author was privileged to join this collective effort in late 1943 and was still working on a WOSB when this book was being written in late 1946. He worked on four Boards and paid working visits to another six or seven. Some techniques here described were developed to their fullest at 10 WOSB (Chester) and 5 WOSB (Wormley, Surrey).

It must be made clear that this book is in no sense official though published with the permission and approval of the Directorate of Army Psychiatry and the War Office. The full official account of WOSB and its statistical validations will no doubt be published in due time. This is an individual reaction to a collective effort; while it derives from a common experience, it includes certain techniques developed locally and not, as yet, adopted as standard basic procedure. The body of techniques here described does however represent what the author considers an optimum pattern of observational field; and he describes only those of which he has intimate knowledge.

Most of these techniques—including those described in Chapter XIX—were in use at Chester about November 1944; what one considered an optimum 3-phase procedure of testing was in use at Wormley by June 1945. The Final Board Profile, described in Chapter XVIII, became standard WOSB procedure in late 1945.

The author was required to observe intensively, for a period of three days, somewhere in the neighbourhood of 6,000 potential officers: of these, upward of 2,500 were interviewed. As there were on an average 8 men to each group, he was given the opportunity of observing approximately 750 groups; each in experimental stress tasks of various kinds.

Special acknowledgements are due to: Col. Guy Hesletine, (Deputy President at Chester, and President at Wormley) for active, continuous co-operation and understanding in experimentation of every kind; to Capt. Ken Murray, Psychological Officer, and Sjts Medcalf and Willet at Chester; to Lt-Col. J. S. Sutherland and the psychological team at the Research and Training Centre at Hampstead and the technical memoranda they produced; to the whole body of WOSB collaborators—controlled by the Directorate of Selection of Personnel on the one hand and the Directorate of Army Psychiatry on the other—too numerous to mention: and especially to Brigadier Torrie—present Director of Army Psychiatry—for every kind of encouragement and help and the opportunity to complete one's researches. Very special acknowledgement is due to Major Gavin Reeve, M.Sc. for his chapter on validation—based on work carried out up to the publication of this book—and for later collaboration of a particularly helpful kind.

The development of WOSB owes much to the inspiration of Dr. J. R. Rees, CBE (lately Brigadier and Consultant in Psychiatry to the Army) who was the catalytic agent in the creative ferment of British Army Psychiatry; it owes also to the constructive and prophetic foresight of Sir Ronald Adam, Bart, GCB, DSO, OBE, lately Adjutant-General, who was responsible for the initiation and fostering of the War Office Selection Board as a psychological and scientific procedure for selecting leaders in the military field.

This book is addressed primarily to those likely to be concerned with selection on leadership or managerial level who have some psychological background. It should have some interest for those who work in the fringing social sciences, for educationalists and for socially-minded people interested in the scientific approach to the study of human relations. It is written as simply as the content permits but even with a psychological background it is doubtful if its full connotations can be appreciated by those who have not witnessed at least one 3-day Board of the type herein described. It must be obvious that psychological techniques cannot be circumscribed in a book but merely adumbrated. The contents of Part I on "Theories", Part III on "Trends" and Chapter XIV are entirely the author's responsibility; they indicate the motives for writing the rest of it.

CHAPTER II

THE FIELD OR GROUP APPROACH IN PSYCHOLOGY

Until 50 years ago, psychology was—as its etymology indicates —the study of the psyche: what the psyche was, no one professed to know and one could only beg that question. But the emphasis was on its cognitive aspect, on thinking and on the intellectual faculties. This approach was comparatively static and sterile and contributed little to human understanding and effort.

With Freud, came a new approach in which the emphasis moved decisively from thinking to feeling; from the processes of thought to the dynamics of emotion; from the conscious content of mind to its total content which included the all-important subconscious realm. It moved from the consideration of static patterns to the analysis and interpretation of dynamic inter-relationships: it began to consider not merely man's conscious appreciation of a situation but his total adjustment to it. This approach was far from sterile and in half a century has fertilised and revolutionised the study of man.

For some years, a new and natural developmental trend in psychology has aimed at relating it to the rest of human ecology. It has aimed at widening the field of enquiry by studying man not as a solitary organism, a unit in vacuo, but as member of a group or community: man in a social field, interacting continuously with the group or groups in which he finds himself: influencing them and being influenced by them.

At this point, where sociology and a psychology—become more social—fringe and fertilise each other, one must distinguish carefully between them: though they cover much the same field, their functions are different. Whereas sociology studies *how* men behave in group situations and *what* they do in these situations, psychology studies *why* man interacts socially as he does and *why* the reactions of the group influence him as they do.

CO-ORDINATING STUDY IN AREA WITH STUDY IN DEPTH

With this widening concept, psychology now seeks to include the dynamics of interpersonal relationships: the *why* as distinct

5

from the *how* of human relations. True, the internal dynamics of Freud—which did consider the social factor especially in the object-relationships of earlier life—still require further development and clarification. But this further development in depth cannot fail to be vastly enriched and helped by the more recent emphasis on man as participating member of a social field. With Freudian study in depth is coordinated the study in social area: psychology becomes neither exclusively individual nor social but a total field which circumscribes and includes and attempts to relate both the field within the individual and the social field i.e. man *and* his group. It follows the threads of interpersonal and intrapersonal dynamics not only vertically into the depths but also laterally into the community. This approach promises to become infinitely more fertile.

The concepts of this "field psychology" have slowly crystallised in the contributions of K. Lewin, J. F. Brown and others: they derive largely from Gestalt psychology and may prove to be critically important and unifying concepts in the history of the human sciences. They may even help towards providing a common discipline for the physical and biological sciences.

The term "field" derives originally from the physics of relativity and connotes a field of related energies as distinct from a structure or pattern which is merely a summation of its parts. It can be illustrated most simply in terms of the Newtonian apple. When this falls from its bough to the ground it does so, not because of any quality residing exclusively in the apple: but —as every student of elementary physics knows—by virtue of a field of forces exerted on the apple: a field of gravitational forces exerted by the earth, the apple and theoretically by every other body in the cosmos. It is the pattern of this gravitational field that determines the apple's motion; and not the qualities of the apple *per se*.

In short, a fundamental axiom of the field approach is that the pattern—or function—of the whole determines the functions of its parts. In Chapter IV—as further extension of this approximation—it will be suggested that the relationship of whole to part is a reciprocal circular dynamic relationship, a simultaneous polarisation of whole and part functions.

In applying this axiom to psychology, one may consider not only social fields or groups but also—as already suggested— fields or dynamic patterns within the individual: both are contained in the total field. But where the field approach attempts to observe the forces within the individual, it can only hope as yet to follow in the wake of the psychoanalytic approach—and well behind. It is in the study of social fields that it promises to make its greatest contributions at the moment: and has—in WOSB technique—already stimulated a major contribution to the study of the leadership function in man.

PERSONALITY AND LEADERSHIP IN TERMS OF THE SOCIAL FIELD

Let us attempt to consider personality and leadership in terms of this approach.

Man is an organism in a field of organisms. As the pattern of the whole determines the functions of its parts, so the social field in which a man finds himself determines the man, his personality and total behaviour (which includes thought and feeling) in that field. The field determines his personality and his personality is a reaction to that field: change the field and you change the man, his personality and his potentialities for achievement and leadership.

In short, if we express the above axiom in terms of the social field, the personality of each member of such a field is a function —in the mathematical sense—of that field: and changes continuously in response to its changing dynamics, its needs, demands, commands, stresses etc.

As a second axiom one would suggest that the development and growth of a personality is the result of its passing inevitably and continuously in space-time from simpler and smaller and fewer fields to larger and more complex and more numerous fields: from the family to the school, the neighbourhood and ultimately into the greater community. Some social fields will inhibit a man's personality in some aspects: others will expand it: all will modify and change it.

As a third axiom one would suggest that in so far as you can choose and control these fields, you may hope to control and influence the personalities in them. Some implications of this axiom for group psychotherapy and sociotherapy, for education and training, will be discussed in Chapters III and XXII.

If man's personality is a function exercised in a social field, his leadership—a measure of his influence on that field—may be regarded as one aspect of that function.

WOSB AND THE GROUP APPROACH

For the words "social field" substitute "group" and you have the key to the rationale of much of WOSB technique.

If one can control under experimental conditions the stresses to which a small group is submitted, one may hope to provide its members both with opportunities for action and leadership and with conditions that limit these opportunities. From their use of these opportunities and their adjustment to these limiting conditions, one may draw tentative estimates of their effectiveness in the group: and these may be related to estimates from other observations and sources.

WOSB used an experimental group of about 8 individuals as testing ground, "micro-community", and experimental social field. Within the framework and context of this group, its members could be submitted in a Leaderless Group or Stress Group Task to varying conditions and stresses: their reactions and inter-actions could be observed, the qualities of their personalities and leadership in that group estimated and a prognosis of likely future development arrived at.

Group techniques of this kind were first formulated—after some experimentation—in May 1942 by the group of psychiatrists and psychologists mentioned in the preface.

From that time, selection in the Army was carried out on two levels and those who became officers were "screened" on both. The fresh recruit was tested on "aptitude" level. A battery of about 8 tests, interviews and a medical and psychological check-up were used to determine the field of activity in which he could be most usefully employed: whether as signaller, gunner infanteer, nursing orderly, clerk, etc.

Personnel Selection Officers earmarked a percentage of these as potential officers. They were instructed to cast their nets widely and to be content if only 50 per cent of their "potentials" eventually proved suitable. Provided general level of intelligence and education were sufficient, personal and leadership qualities could be estimated later at WOSB. Within three months of entering the Army, these potential officers were sent to a WOSB to be "screened" for OCTU (Officer Cadet Training Unit): along with any others whom the units considered might make the grade. Most of the latter had not been through selection procedure on aptitude level but there might be one or two who had impressed the unit more than they had impressed the PSO.

WOSBs were scattered all over the country, usually in country houses: and there, candidates lived under officer conditions for 3 days while being observed and tested on leadership —not aptitude—level. The emphasis now was not on a man's aptitudes or primarily on his technical capacity—though that would be considered—but on the quality of his personality in a social field and on his ability to manage men in the field of activity for which he was being considered.

CHAPTER III

THE GROUP

Under the influence of the "field" approach, psychology is interesting itself more and more in man as an individual functioning in a group: in the dynamics of his interactions *with*—and his influence *on*—the group.

The group looms so large in WOSB technique and in this book that one might profitably at this stage mobilise such knowledge and ideas as one has. One's approach as a psychotherapist come to selection *via* group-psychotherapy—and other reasons that will unfold themselves—have determined the headings under which we will now discuss the group.

OFFICER SELECTION IN TERMS OF THE GROUP

In popular terms, selection means putting the square peg into the square hole. In more dynamic terms it may be defined as putting a man into a group and into a field of activity where he can function happily and efficiently on his optimum level of efficiency to the advantage of himself and the group.

Common experience suggests that a man—however stable—may fail to adjust to a completely unsuitable group: whereas another more limited and less stable, demoralised man may—in a carefully selected group—adjust and contribute increasingly well. The well-chosen group will tend to de-condition any "vicious circles" he has got into: and to condition a "virtuous circle" by which he will gradually normalise himself.

How then select the right man for the right group?

WOSB's answer was to test and evaluate him in the context of the small experimental group submitted to considerable time and problem stress i.e. required to execute a difficult task against time.

That which one sought to observe and evaluate one might call his group-effectiveness, the sum-total of his contribution to the group and its task. In this book, we will differentiate group-effectiveness into the following components:—

    1 the effective *level of his functioning:* of his ability to contribute towards the functional aspect of the common task by

planning and organising the available abilities, materials, time, etc.

2 his *group-cohesiveness* or ability to bind the group in the direction of the common task: to relate its members emotionally to each other and to the task.

3 his *stability* or ability to stand up to resistances and frustrations without serious impairment of (1) or (2) and the results of their interplay.

In short, in the WOSB technique of officer selection, one observes a man *in* a group-task in order to determine his group-effectiveness (in a particular field): one selects and *tests* him *in* a group *for* a group.

NEUROSIS IN TERMS OF THE GROUP

In psychotherapy, on the other hand, one *trains* and prepares the maladjusted individual for the group i.e. the larger group or community: in group therapy indeed, one trains and rehabilitates him *in* a group *for* the group. The medical psychologist has therefore something to contribute to the group approach.

More and more it is becoming apparent to the psychotherapist that his function is to break the vicious circle of neurosis that isolates a man from the community and to help him back to his right level and right field in that community. The neurotic has lost his group and does not know where to find it: it is the psychotherapist's job to help him find it. The neurotic is a demoralised man: psychosis is the utter fragmentation of the personality that ensues with completest demoralisation.

Starved of the deep-seated organic satisfactions that can come only from the group, his wild, aimless, neurotically compulsive strivings to be accepted by the group—based on no warm understanding of it—can lead only to a vicious circle of needless suffering. Ignorant of the natural way he perforce must drive himself the difficult way. His compulsive straining to recover his morale bankrupts his reserves of energy and induces instability. His neurosis is, at one and the same time, a compulsive attempt to restore his group-effectiveness and the suffering of being unable to do so. Even if talent or genius result occasionally as a by-product of that suffering and striving and enable him to work on a high functional level, the cost in energy must lead to a gross diminishment of his stability and capacity for a normal *joie de vivre*.

In short, neurosis is a vicious circle in which faulty and

immature social attitudes lead to some degree of removal from the group: this to a diminished group-effectiveness despite greater effort and to a lessening of stability: finally to a gradual deterioration in social attitudes which feeds the vicious circle of increasing isolation, ineffectiveness and unhappiness.

THE CAUSES OF NEUROSIS IN TERMS OF THE GROUP

What are the causes of this vicious circle?

Some of the factors *seem* to operate predominantly from within outwards i.e. from individual dispositions: others from without in, from the social environment and the group. Let us call the former centrifugal and the latter centripetal.

Common centrifugal factors are the faulty early object-relationships of childhood. Psychoanalytic investigation in depth has revealed how these—if uncorrected—develop into faulty adult object-relationships and interpersonal attitudes. To take two examples, slightly schematised.

The life of one man will be dominated by resentment of the father figure which he sees in all authority good or bad. The leitmotif of his life—largely not conscious—is the desire to punish, dominate, surpass and compel admiration from that figure.

The life of another will be permeated by an excessive emotional dependence on the mother figure, which leads him to expect and demand an excessive display of affection from all. His ambivalent attitude to the mother figure makes him resent—and at the same time, crave—the source of this affection which he cannot command at will.

Both of these attitudes in the adult must tend to deprive him of the rewards and satisfactions of the group and to initiate the vicious circle of isolation, demoralisation and neurosis.

Centripetal factors are too many to list: but we may mention a few. The community may create anxiety in a man by giving him a job that is too big; or frustration by a job that is too small. It may condemn a man of high intelligence to work which makes excessive demands on his weaknesses and insufficient or none on his strengths: so that frustration leads to resentment, restlessness and increasing isolation.

It can, by the same token, break the vicious circle of isolation and demoralisation by employing him, within his diminished capacity on a lower level or in another field and so bringing him "into the picture": or by crediting him with a modicum of

approval and sanction before these have been earned. It can ease
the strain on poor social attitudes by choosing a setting which
makes few or no demands on them. Neurosis is relative to the
task: and if you compel a man to keep attempting a job to which
he is unequal, eventually you make a neurotic of him.

THE TREATMENT AND PREVENTION OF NEUROSIS IN TERMS OF THE GROUP

The causes of a vicious circle operate usually not at any one
point in the circle but at a number of points in its circumference.
Perhaps the spiral is a more graphic symbol of the accumulative
effects of such causes: the downward "vicious spiral" and the
upward "virtuous spiral" if one cares to adopt that symbolic
convention.

To reverse the vicious spiral of neurotic adjustment, therapy
will need to operate simultaneously at as many points in the
spiral as possible. We will schematically isolate three of these
phases to correspond with the three aspects of group-effectiveness
mentioned above. These are:—

1 a diminished level of functioning:
2 faulty interpersonal relationships that either disrupt the
   group, fail to "bind" it or even lead to isolation:
3 diminished stability or capacity for work in relation to its
   level, tempo, duration or other stresses specific to the job.

Of these, the first and third may be influenced predominantly
through centripetal factors, the second through centrifugal
factors by individual or group psychotherapy. The latter will
attempt to give the neurotic insight into the defective social
attitudes that are isolating him: the former will relieve him of
some of the strain while he re-orientates and stabilises himself.

The psychotherapist is beginning to realise that his is a double
function: *on the one hand to help the individual cope with the community,
on the other hand to help the community cope with the individual.*

In so far as he influences the individual via the community,
he may do this in two ways: in a more direct short-term approach
i.e. some sort of sociotherapy; or in a less direct long-term
approach i.e. some sort of "sociatry".

In sociotherapy, he attempts immediate modifications of the
neurotic's social field. With the help of social workers and other
collaborators he may influence, modify or change the job,

responsibilities, conditions at home, school, work etc. The strain may be eased by diminishing the volume, tempo or level of his work: by partial or complete rest or hospitalisation where necessary. Selection—on either aptitude or leadership level—is perhaps a major form of sociotherapy for the "complex 25 per cent" of the community; and of constructive social medicine for the remaining 75 per cent.

In "sociatry" (derived by analogy from "psychiatry": I am not fond of either word), what is attempted is a long-term modification of the basic institutions of society itself. *Just as the psychotherapist attempts to diagnose and correct faulty attitudes of the individual towards the community, so the sociatrist will attempt to diagnose and correct faulty attitudes of the community towards its members.*

The word is as tentative as the idea. The medical psychologist is more aware of sociatric implications than most because he cannot escape being reminded of them by his patients. But he is only one of the many who will exercise such a function: no doubt a wider sociatric awareness will diffuse throughout the community to all capable of exercising some constructive influence.

In so far as the psychotherapist influences the individual directly he may do so in individual or group therapy or a co-ordination of both. To any form of psychotherapy, he will of course add the full resources of the physician's armamentarium. Not least valuable will be his ability to "cotton-wool" the patient temporarily against excessive stress by the controlled and tactical use of sedative drugs.

The therapeutic interview of individual psychotherapy is essentially a "stress interview" in which the patient is compelled to face the unpleasant facts on various levels of his personality; and is induced to develop insight into them. With insight, it is hoped that he will abandon the ineffective social roles—based on unhealthy object-relationships and muddled phantasy thinking—that he has been vainly attempting to enact: and will accept and master roles for which he is more suitable, which are in themselves more mature and which should ultimately increase his effectiveness and zest.

SOME EXPERIMENTS IN GROUP-THERAPY AND GROUP-REHABILITATION

Experiments in group-therapy and group-analysis first aimed to save psychotherapeutic man-hours in order to provide even

a superficial psychotherapy for more people. Still later, the value
of projecting interpersonal attitudes within the group and of
linking the relatively isolated individual with the group was
realised. The likelihood is that both individual and group
therapy have their specific uses and can be successfully combined
and co-ordinated.

An early experiment in group analysis—which I was able to
observe in 1935 and 1936—was made by Schilder at the New
York Bellevue Psychopathic Hospital Out-patients Department.
About 6–8 male patients were treated in a small group. All had
one or more individual interviews before being inducted into
the group: some were given occasional individual interviews
subsequently. Into this "micro-community" they were allowed
and encouraged to project and develop their habitual interpersonal attitudes towards the rest of the group. The nature of
these attitudes became increasingly apparent after a few sessions:
and by discussion and mutual criticism—with the catalytic help
of the therapist—and by analysing these attitudes as they actually
arose, each was helped to further insight. It was easier to note
faulty attitudes in oneself after one had noted them in others:
and attitudes projected and revealed in action could be modified
in action.

The attempt was made to analyse interpersonal attitudes in
terms of a Freud-derived "depth" psychology. Few, if any,
subsequent experiments in group-therapy seem to have attempted
so deep an analysis. The essence of the experiment however was
to encourage the individual to project and solve his problems
in a group of individuals with similar problems: to develop—
in the framework of the "micro-community"—new insights,
social attitudes and techniques which might gradually be extended
into the "macro-community."

In an experiment by Bion and Rickman at Northfields
Military Hospital in 1943, groups of patients were engaged in
work projects which compelled them to accept and tolerate and
deal with the psychological limitations of others as well as of
themselves.

Because of the uncooperativeness of some and their difficulty
in fitting into group activities the group as a whole was
stimulated:—

a to deal constructively with that uncooperativeness,

b later, to become aware individually of its manifestations in themselves and to cope with these.

The experiment was calculated to lead them to the realisation that neurosis is closely associated with faulty social attitudes and that only by modifying these and regaining a sane relationship to society, can neurotic adjustment give way to a healthy social adjustment.

Though Northfields technique aimed to produce insight at a more superficial layer of consciousness than Schilder's group-analysis, it achieved a closer relationship to reality in the work project. At a later stage, Northfields based its therapy on "depth" psychology.

An important later development of the group approach was made by Wilson, Trist and Rodger in 1945 at the Civil Rehabilitation Units organised by the British Army for ex-prisoners-of-war.

Its importance lay in this: that it was not therapeutic or corrective but an actual attempt to help men coming from one social field to adjust to a vastly different one, via the transitional community of the CRU where they spent 4 weeks or more.

As soldiers in captivity, they had spent years in that rigid, inhibited group-life with its limited social locomotions, its acquired habit of resenting authority and of non-cooperation with it. They were now required to adjust to a freer civilian life whose opportunities and demands for spontaneity and free social locomotion; whose need for frequent decisions on trivial matters instead of a passive obeying of instructions; and whose need for cooperation with authority on all levels at first tended to arouse acute anxiety. An anxiety which they often related to anything but its true causes i.e. the conflict between acquired habit and present necessity. Those who had been captive for more than 2 years experienced definite neurotic difficulties—often with little insight—which benefited even from mild group-therapy at the CRU.

Psychologically, these men required the adroit balancing of inducements to social initiative and increasing self-help with a slow tactful withdrawal of the initial emotional support given them. When left to fend for themselves—in their unwillingness to make decisions—they clamoured for measures of control and discipline but these were resisted by the staff. Everything was planned to encourage them to use spontaneously the facilities available and to make their own programmes, preferably in groups of their own formation: nothing was compulsory except pay parade.

Some visited factories and workshops and made exploratory trips into the possibilities of civilian life: others brushed up their skills in work-shops and studios: still others attended Brains Trusts by industrial and other experts.

All were encouraged—but no pressure was exerted—to discuss their domestic, health and vocational problems with social workers, vocational psychologists, Ministry of Labour representatives, physicians, psychiatrists etc. The psychiatrist encouraged those who consulted him—and the obviously maladjusted who did not—to discuss their problems in small groups so that they might gain insight and reassurance from others with similar problems and reactions.

An interesting aspect of the experiment was the opportunity it gave to observe the reactions of members of the social field to which the ex-captive was returning i.e. employers, fellow-workers, wives, children etc. It called attention too, to the sort of tensions and anxieties that arise when men and communities are presented with wider opportunities for free democratic self-government and are required on relatively short notice to assume a much greater measure of social initiative and responsibility than hitherto.

THE COORDINATION OF SELECTION AND MEDICAL PSYCHOLOGY IN THE ARMY

Selection aims at testing a man's group-effectiveness to determine his position in the community: the medical psychologist aims at correcting or preventing attitudes that diminish his group-effectiveness and personal happiness. In so far as he aims to prevent maladjustment, he can contribute usefully by assisting the selector in the placement of the "complex 25 per cent" of the population in jobs that will tend to stabilise them.

The British Army in wartime provided an effective large-scale coordination of the work of Personnel Selection Officers and medical psychologists; not only at all stages of selection but also in the rehabilitation of men hospitalised for psychiatric breakdowns and in the re-allocation of men subjected to years of captivity as prisoner-of-war.

At Primary Training Centres, where recruits spent their first

6 weeks, PSO and medical psychologist worked hand in hand in selection on "aptitude"—rather than "leadership"—level. After a battery of tests, medical examinations and interviews, the men were "screened" for the medical psychologist who interviewed on an average about 12–15 per cent of them, recommending some for specific jobs and others for treatment or discharge. Those earmarked as potential officers by the PSO came to WOSB about 3 months later to pass an even more intensive psychological screening to ensure that none undertook officer responsibility who might break down under it.

A later screening took place at Army Selection Centres which dealt with (1) those whose first placement by the PTC had proved unsuitable; (2) those whose change of medical category necessitated a change of job; (3) NCOs who required a change of job for any reason. All were screened for the medical psychologist who saw—and advised on—a percentage of them.

Armies prepared for the desert campaign in North Africa and for the liberation of France underwent a complete selection procedure which included all soldiers enlisted in pre-selection days. Apart from any effect on efficiency and morale, this seems to have reduced the incidence of psychiatric casualties.

An "annexure" scheme was adopted at military psychiatric hospitals for men recovered from a psychiatric breakdown who would ordinarily have been discharged and lost to the Army. These men were posted to specific jobs—considered within their powers and likely to stabilise them—from which they could not be posted without special permission from War Office. This follow-up of therapy by special posting seems to have been successful from the viewpoint of both Army and the individual.

Prisoners-of-war—released in large numbers in 1945—were also passed through a selection screen, by PSOs and medical psychologists, before being either discharged or trained for other duties.

CHAPTER IV

THE LEADER

A PRELIMINARY DEFINITION OF LEADERSHIP

Without daring to attempt a preciser definition at this stage, one may suggest provisionally that leadership is the measure and degree of an individual's ability to influence—and be influenced by—a group in the implementation of a common task. This circumscribes three important aspects of leadership function: the individual, the group and the task: and indicates leadership as a functional relationship between these three basic variables.

In respect of the first two, it can only be highly effective if based on a sensitive understanding of the group's needs and on the ability to be influenced by it. The leader who dominates and drives a group towards an end they do not seek is unlikely to retain his leadership: his domination is brittle and will stand little stress. In so far as he considers the needs and mobilises the initiative of every member in the group: in so far as he helps them towards the goal which will give the group its greatest satisfaction and provide every member of it with the profound gratification of effective participation on his own level and at his own optimum tempo. In so far as he does these things, his leadership is more real, more flexible, more resistant to stress and incidentally more democratic—in the better sense of that word—than any leadership which is insensitive to the group in which it is exercised.

In so far as he does these things, he shows leadership *and* followership: these are reciprocal but not inverse qualities of the leader. In any group which is reacting and interacting to effect a common purpose, it is never correct to say that one man does all the leading and the others all the following. Leadership and followership are working relationships between men on a job which concerns them all. The better leader knows when to follow and whom: when to influence and when to be influenced: when to direct and when to accept direction: when—in analytic terms— to identify himself with the good benign father in relation to the group and when with the respectful son.

In Chapter II, we considered as an axiom of field psychology, that the pattern or function of the whole determines the functions of its parts. It might be truer to say that a field is a polarisation of the whole and its parts: that a group and its members are reciprocally and dynamically related in a polarised circular relationship. There is no need to assume either to be a prime or antecedent cause: in any circular relationship—such as exists in a "field", Gestalt or dynamic pattern—the temporal or chronological relationship of cause and effect hardly seems to be relevant. In a space-time continuum, causality cannot be confined to the coordinate of time alone. Member and group interact to influence each other simultaneously and continuously: leadership is one aspect of that interaction, followership another. At any moment, both leadership and followership function derive simultaneously from the whole group and from every member of it: it is a collective and simultaneous relationship.

LEADERSHIP A SERIES—NOT A DICHOTOMY

A dangerous fallacy is the dichotomy of mankind into leaders and non-leaders. Each one of us exercises some influence on our community on some level and in some field: and that influence —however little—is the measure of our leadership: our contribution to the collective effort and to the collective leadership of the group.

A man's functional position in the social field at any moment is fixed by the two coordinates of level of function and field of activity.

Let us consider "level" first.

Field psychology has rightly emphasised the fallacies inherent in a false dichotomy. Leadership—as the ability to exercise influence on the group—is not a dichotomy but a continuous series.

If you rank a hundred men in order of height—from the tallest to the shortest—at what stage can you say this man is tall but his neighbour is short? Height is here a continuous series, not a dichotomy. If you rank similarly on intelligence (as measured by "intelligence tests") at what point can you say this man is stupid but his neighbour is intelligent?

The fallacy of a false dichotomy has crept, more insidiously and dangerously, into the field of medicine in the commonly held concepts of the sick and healthy: the normal and the abnormal: the neurotic and the stable. The resultant confusion

may easily hamper the efforts of social and constructive medicine.
In the field of medical psychology, it becomes increasingly
obvious that it is profitable to consider a man's mental health
in terms not of the abnormal or normal but of his capacity to
adjust happily and effectively to the demands of the community
and life generally at a given moment. Arrange the same series
of a hundred men in the order of their capacity to adjust effectively to life (if one could easily rank a series of that sort) and at
what stage can you say: this man is normal but his neighbour is
abnormal? Even if you eliminate as abnormal those who have
broken down (and they may recover), or those who are having
considerable difficulty in adjusting and are undergoing much
suffering, at what degree of suffering or difficulty will you say
that a man ceases to be abnormal or neurotic? It is true of course
that if you hospitalise a man you create a temporary dichotomy
of the down-bedded and the upstanding.

Leadership—like adjustment; like most dynamic functions of
man in the social field—is probably considered more profitably
in terms of a continuous series rather than of an arbitrary dichotomy: there is no warrant for the assumption that it emerges at
a certain fixed point in the series. One must keep in mind however
that it is exercised in a variety of fields; and that leadership level
is therefore never a *point* in that series but a *range* of function.

As a continuous series—and not a dichotomy of leaders and
non-leaders—it still becomes necessary to decide what level and
upwards constitutes officership: that level cannot be fixed but
will be relative to the demands of the situation and the supply of
men. If, out of a hundred men, ten officers are required, they
will be taken naturally from the 91st percentile upwards in the
leadership series. If however the exigencies of the situation
demand 15 officers, then officership will be invested from the
86th percentile upwards: those from the 86th to the 90th percentile
will either be—or not be—officers according to the demand. It
is therefore not correct to say—as has on occasion been said—
that a man is either an officer or not: nor is there anything to
warrant the assumption that officership emerges at a certain fixed
point in the series. The arbitrary level which separates the
officer from the "other-rank" may—and does—change with the
demand. That men are accepted as emergency officers who
would not be accepted as regulars indicates that the level is
considered to be relative. Indeed we need not take it for granted

that the conventional and nominal and artificial dichotomy into officer and "other-rank" is the most efficient or most democratic method of ranking in military or other fields.

LEVEL OF LEADERSHIP VARIES WITH THE FIELD

Leadership being a functional relationship between a group, its members and a task, let us consider the task or field of activity.

Incidentally the term "field" is used here with three different connotations which the context will clarify:

1 the entire social field i.e. member plus rest of group plus task:
2 the field of activity i.e. task or type of task alone:
3 the observational field or pattern of tests in which men and group are observed i.e. the WOSB 3-phase pattern.

As a simple example of leadership in terms of field activity, imagine a small community stranded on a remote uninhabited island. If there is a doctor in the group, he will tend to assume leadership in matters of health and hygiene: a carpenter, builder or engineer if there is need for building or construction: a soldier will take charge if hostile natives appear. The group may—and will—choose different leaders for its different purposes: yet, by the same token, one or more members of that group will tend to assume a general leadership of the group which will be accepted by all; including those whose leadership in certain specific fields is unquestioned.

What is the nature of that general leadership and how is it related to leadership in specific fields?

ARE THERE G FACTORS IN LEADERSHIP?

Are there g factors in leadership which determine general level in all fields? Are there s factors which influence and modify that general level only in specific fields i.e. in relation to certain tasks?

Is leadership a composite of g and s factors so that one might make the formulation: $L = g + s$ (where L = leadership level in a certain field, g = influence of the g factors and s = the modifying influence of the s factors in that field)?

To polarise our speculations from the general with observations from the particular, it is evident even in military fields—

when choosing officers for Infantry, RAPC, RASC, RAC, RE, REME, etc.—that special factors do play some part. In Infantry, for instance, general factors seem to be more important in the face-to-face leadership required: in REME or RAPC, it seems evident that less of these general factors may be compensated for—to some extent—by greater skill, technical experience or a strong identification with that particular field of activity. No doubt these can never fully compensate for a low level in the general factors: but it seems common experience—to those who have helped to select officers—that where general factors in leadership are borderline, special factors may bring it up to officer level and are therefore determinant in those cases.

It is too early to attempt a clear formulation of the nature of leadership. Provisionally and tentatively one will suggest that the whole of leadership (including both g and s factors) may be represented by the concept of "group-effectiveness" with its 3 components (a) level of functioning (b) group-cohesiveness and (c) stability.

Of these, g factors may be considered to determine (b) and part of (a) i.e. a minimal range of intelligence and education. (One's own investigations—as yet unpublished—indicate that a large percentage of those who break down as officers have a level of intelligence and education which is low as compared with the general run of officers).

The s factors may be considered to determine the remainder of (a) i.e. certain *special aptitudes* and also specific *attitudes to the field of activity* (the degree to which the individual is identified with that activity and interests allied to it).

Both g and s factors will condition (c).

Whether it eventually becomes possible or desirable to consider general and special factors in leadership, the existence of general factors—and the relative importance of group-cohesiveness in the general pattern of leadership function—was tacitly assumed in WOSB practice. That special factors might be determinant—especially in the more technical arms—was also generally accepted: or at any rate acted upon.

s FACTORS IN LEADERSHIP

The s factors, i.e. special aptitudes and attitudes, are best investigated in technical interviews and examinations; in special aptitude tests; in an evaluation of Spearmans s factors (verbal,

B

spatial, etc.) in specially weighted intelligence tests; in investigations of special interests and attitudes by "projective" techniques.

WOSB made an extremely interesting experimental investigation (Chapter XII) into "engineering personality" for the purpose of selecting schoolboys to be trained for technical commissions in the Army or for engineering posts in civil life. "Apparatus sessions" were used in which the attitudes to—and ability with—apparatus of various kinds were noticed: there were also interest quizzes and talks to obtain an impression of the candidates' trends. Investigations of this type promise to be of special value in modifying WOSB technique for selection in other professional or technical fields.

In Stress Group Tasks, while the *difficulty of the task* helps to reveal the general level of group-effectiveness, the *nature of the task*—discussion, practical, planning, etc.—may reveal some of the s factors.

But with all these considerations of g and s factors, one must still remember that no two fields or situations or tasks are ever the same: that no man's emotional and physical and social attributes ever remain fixed on one level: that leadership is a dynamic and adaptive function, varying with both the group and the task, waxing and waning with the demands of the total situation, fluctuating in time. Despite these considerations it was still possible in WOSB practice to obtain an estimate of probable average level that was sufficiently useful.

LEADERSHIP AS AN ATTRIBUTE OF THE HEALTHY PERSONALITY

What seems to emerge is that every man should be capable of some degree of leadership—influencing others towards a satisfying participation in collective effort; and being sensitive to the influence of others—on his own level and in his own field of activity: and one might regard it as a basic sign of mental and social health that he show some degree of effective, happy and spontaneous leadership on that level. In that sense, every man should be a leader.

To the selector, the sample of group-effectiveness revealed in a Stress Group Task points to the quality and level of a man's leadership. To the medical psychologist, observing the same task, it will point to the extent to which he has developed sufficiently healthy interpersonal attitudes to participate fully in the group's work and so to fulfil his potentialities for leadership and zestful living. If these interpersonal attitudes are unhealthy and inadequate, he will adjust poorly: and if they lead to a serious weakening of his bonds with the group which may ultimately isolate him from it, he is on the way to neurosis—or psychosis.

Leadership then may be regarded as the expression of a man's adequately realised group-effectiveness on his own natural level: neurosis as the indication and result of an inadequately realised group-effectiveness; of some impediment (be it external, internal or both) in the realisation of his potential group-effectiveness, natural leadership and capacity for zestful living.

It should hardly be necessary to point out that to be a participating member of a group is not antithetical to one's individuality in that group. To be individual is necessarily to be different in many ways: and one can only be different if one has something to be different *from*: and some place and some audience to be different *in* and *with*. Far from an antithesis between participation and individuality, they are interdependent; and without that interdependent relationship, there *can* be no individuality.

CHAPTER V

THE LEADERLESS GROUP OR STRESS GROUP TASK

I—WHAT IT IS

ITS RATIONALE

WOSB submits a man to varying time, problem and social stresses in an experimental "micro-community" of about 8 members, committed to tasks of different types i.e. outdoor physical, indoor planning, group discussion etc. No leader is appointed and the group is allowed to throw up its own natural leaders. From observation of the man's group-effectiveness in several different activities under varying degrees of stress it gains a balanced impression of his general group-effectiveness which it checks and co-ordinates with tests of him as an individual either *apart* from the group or in charge of it. Coordinating group tests with individual tests is an important technical device in WOSB.

By varying in this way the field of activity and the degree of stress in the group task, one may draw conclusions about the man's ability in various fields, his "contact" with people and the amount of stress he can tolerate without serious deterioration of his effectiveness.

Eight was found to be the optimum number for the experimental group: partly because it was the largest number which put no excessive strain on the observers' span of attention: partly because a lesser number would have provided insufficient "stooge" material for those in the group with some leadership.

ITS SOURCES

The Leaderless Group—as this technique was named—was worked out by Bion, Sutherland, Trist and a team of Army psychiatrists and psychologists. It derives from several sources.

In 1941 J. R. P. French of USA had reported an experimental study of the emotional behaviour of organised and unorganised (i.e. leaderless) groups in extreme frustration produced by requiring them to solve insoluble problems which they were led to believe were soluble. The concept of using the experimental group as a testing environment derives very naturally from the field approach in psychology: if man is an organism functioning in a social field, then his social functions are best observed in that field: in a group which may be natural (i.e. uncontrolled) or experimental (i.e. controlled).

Another source of the "leaderless" concept is the "free association" of ordinary analytic therapy and especially its group variant as practised by Schilder, etc. In "free association" one encourages the patient to utter whatever comes to mind spontaneously and freely: in the expectation that sooner or later he will say something significant which may project and reveal to the skilled interpreter—and later to himself—the pattern or leitmotif of his life or some of the threads thereof. A group encouraged to behave spontaneously will sooner or later reveal each man as he is in relation to that group. In children, the opportunity might be provided in group play: in the adult, work is the more natural excuse for group activity. The very urgency of the stressful occasions to which the group is submitted will tend to compel spontaneity on that particular level of effort.

Stress is implicit in the Leaderless Group task as in the psychotherapeutic session: in the former it is induced by the task, in the latter by the therapist's insistence that the patient continue to face and discuss topics so painful or unpleasant that he would gladly skim them by. In the analytic group session—as practised by Schilder—the group were similarly compelled to face the stressful task of realising and modifying some of their emotional and social attitudes. This type of session became a sort of Stress Group Task.

ITS NAME

Perhaps the Leaderless Group too might better be described as a Stress Group Task. "Leaderless Group" is intended to indicate that no leader is initially chosen but might imply that none ever arises.

The words "leader" and "leadership" were not much favoured in WOSB and might be sparsely used in selection:—

a because of their looseness of connotation (they imply so many things to so many people, i.e. the ability to dominate, bully, persuade, plan, teach, administrate, etc).

    b because they carry the connotation of a dichotomy of
      leaders and followers rather than the concept of a con-
      tinuous series.
    c because they connote the overt dominance of the type
      found in the "pecking orders" of the zoological kingdom
      (the order of dominance in which chickens, monkeys,
      etc. tend to rank themselves): whereas overt dominance
      —it will be contended here—is of ever-decreasing signi-
      ficance in the higher levels of leadership.

Possibly a more fruitful, less inhibiting concept than "leadership" would be "Group-effectiveness" which one might consider
as being exercised on any level.

A possible objection to "Stress Group Task"—not a serious
one—is that it may. lead some fractionally informed people to
surmise it to be a painful and Gestapo-like procedure. It would
of course not be used before candidates.

ITS VARIETIES AND THEIR COORDINATION

The Leaderless Group is unorganised (has no appointed
leaders) but may—as regards its task—be directed or undirected.

In the WOSB Group Discussion—an indoor task involving
the management of men and ideas—the discussion is usually
undirected, i.e. no topic is set but the conversation is allowed to
follow its own spontaneous directions. The session can be considerably improved by directing the last part of it: if, after 45
minutes of undirected discussion, a highly provocative topic of
general interest—an emotional bomb—is tossed into the group
for 10–15 minutes vivid high-tempo discussion.

The WOSB Progressive Group Task—an outdoor task involving the management of men and materials—is unorganised
but directed. The task includes several sub-tasks or obstacles of
progressive difficulty and increasing frustration. Tasks will
naturally be related to the field of activity for which men are
being selected. If they are to be soldiers, the testing pattern may
include physical outdoor tasks though these are not indispensable
or even necessary: if they are to be civil servants, group discussions or planning projects will be more relevant.

In the WOSB 3-phase procedure here described, the first
phase or Basic Series consists of a Group Discussion followed by
a Progressive Group Task which together gives a balanced

impression of the candidates' group-effectiveness in relation to men, materials and ideas. The third phase is usually another confirmatory Progressive Group Task.

The Planning Project consists of 2 parts:

1 an individual planning phase
2 a Leaderless Group phase (unorganised but directed) in which the candidates meet in committee—without chairman—to organise their plans.

The Human Problems Session has a Leaderless Group background into which other types of grouping are interwoven.

II—WHAT IT MAY REVEAL

GROUP-EFFECTIVENESS

1—*Its Three Aspects*

In Chapter III, we differentiated group-effectiveness into:

a ability in the purely functional aspect of the job
b group-cohesiveness or ability in the social aspect
c stability.

It is important to distinguish clearly between (a) and (b): simple when realised but not always realised. One man may do little yet assist group-cohesion and the group's effectiveness: another may do—or seem to do—much, yet his essential selfishness and egocentricity is such that it eventually disrupts the group's efforts.

So important did WOSB consider (b) that for a time it designated (a) as the "pseudo-task" and (b) as the "real task" and suggested that the observer, while seeming to observe (a) was really focusing on (b). While seemingly observing the set task (i.e. crossing obstacles or keeping a discussion going—on which the candidate was concentrating), he was really noting his ability to assist group-cohesion.

However the ability to plan and organise and the ability to bind and persuade the group in the direction of the plan are so inevitably inter-related in the total task that there seems little point in calling one "real" and the other "pseudo". It seems however to be true that in a relatively short selection procedure, one is likelier to get a sample of "contact" than of "level".

2—To What Extent is Each Revealed?

The Stress Group Task may not throw equal light on each of these aspects.

One cannot be sure of getting an adequate sample of a man's true "level" in the time. He may be prevented from indicating it by immaturity, undue modesty, anxiety, being overshadowed by more dominant or more efficient or more experienced members of the group, etc. Naturally the more efficient the testing technique, the better the sample.

One must keep in mind too that "level" varies appreciably from one field of activity to another: hence the balancing of practical activities with abstract planning and discussion, as in the Basic Series. One must also relate this impression to the paper-screening, the PSO battery of tests, the interviews, etc. If his apparent level does not correspond sufficiently to his potential level (as indicated by intelligence, education, etc.) one must ask oneself why?

The task should always give a reasonably good projection of the candidate's group-cohesiveness. This can be further clarified in the Human Problems Session, which is to the Stress Group Task as the fine adjustment of a microscope to the coarse: it pinpoints a query area in the candidate's social personality in order to gain critical information about that area.

The diagnosis of stability from behaviour in the group is largely a matter for the psychiatrist assisted by the psychologist. But there are many reactions to frustration—at the impasses or critically stressful moments—which observers may be taught to note for referral to the psychiatrist for his interpretation.

In brief, the Stress Group Task throws most light on group-cohesiveness: it should in a balanced pattern of tasks give a useful sample of actual level and suggest possible reasons for failure to realise potential level: it may provide samples of morale and pointers to stability from his frustration reactions to the impasses.

GROUP-COHESIVENESS

A group task demands of each member that he reconcile his personal ambitions and desire to shine with the demands of the group: the desire to do well for himself with the desire to make a useful and appreciated contribution.

In so far as he can solve this conflict constructively, his activities are *group-cohesive* and will help to (a) relate the group emotionally to each other (b) relate them emotionally to the common task: he will bind them as a group and get them identified with the task.

In so far as he fails to do the former, he will be either *group-disruptive* or *group-dependent* (merging into the "isolate" who has no emotional contact with the group and neither gives nor gets). These 3 types—as projected in the Stress Group Task—will be considered again in this chapter and in Chapters x and xiv.

The latter ability (to relate them *emotionally* to the common task, to "bring them into the picture") must be distinguished from the ability to relate them *functionally* to it in terms of their capacities and skills. This is part of the organising phase of functional level (specifically the allocation of men to jobs) and will be discussed as such below.

LEVEL OF FUNCTIONING AND ITS PHASES

T. E. Coffin in "A Three-Component Theory of Leadership" (Journ. Abn. Soc. Psych. vol. 39, p. 63–83; June 1944) considers leadership in terms of 3 phases or roles i.e. planning, organising and persuasion.

Planning deals with the determination of *aims and objectives:* what are the specific problems to be solved and what are their solutions? Organising deals with *ways and means:* with the organising, coordinating and control of people and materials in relation to functions, time, space, etc. Persuasion corresponds largely to what we have called group-cohesiveness.

Psychologically, planning is a first differentiation of the total situation into its primary demands and their solutions: an appreciation of the total situation in its widest terms and the determining of the aims and objectives likely to meet it: a formulation of the query to be answered and of the answer to it in general terms.

Organising may be regarded as a further differentiation of the Gestalt—a breaking down of the total situation—into its sub-tasks and their solutions. It is concerned therefore with ways and means of implementing the aims and objectives of the planning phase. Specifically it concerns itself with such things as: sub-planning generally, the assignment of special jobs and functions to specific people, delegation and control on all levels; the allocation of materials, listing of priorities, elimination of "red herrings", the mechanics of time and motion study etc. In designing tests of

B*

the Planning Project type, points such as these must be kept in mind.

In so far as organising deals with materials in space, it will design: with activities in time, it will draw up programmes and schedules: in wedding people to jobs, it will create functions and functional inter-relationships and the sanctions, authorities and responsibilities that go with them. In so far as it allows for the inevitable flux in events and anticipates some of its possible directions, it will devise procedures for reconsidering the changing situation and creating new functional relationships between men and their jobs and each other wherever the present solution reveals its inadequacy. It should not wait for crisis or acute conflict to reveal this but should anticipate it.

With regard to "persuasion" (Coffin's third phase) one's own tendency at the moment is to dissociate a man's functional contribution to the common task from his social or group-cohesive contribution. One prefers to postulate the functional contribution as operating on 3 levels, phases or roles, 1 planning 2 organising, 3 practical execution: and to regard the social contribution (i.e. "persuasion") as one that may be exercised—to reinforce the functional contribution—at any level or phase from planning to execution, from idea to performance. The planning and the persuading are different aspects of leadership: not different levels of it.

As one passes from planning—through organising—to the practical execution of the job, it still becomes necessary to improvise *ad hoc* minute-to-minute solutions for *ad hoc* problems: to iron out problems as they arise at the immediate impact of effort with reality. There is still need for the exercise of influence and leadership: in few fields of activity can leadership cease where action begins. One cannot exclude from the function of leadership such sub-functions as instruction, demonstration, example, correction, supervision, some aspects of control, etc. In short we must still think of leadership as a series and not as a dichotomy. At the bottom of that series is such simple leadership as the giving of general (i.e. military) commands or drill.

As one descends from planning through organising to practical execution, the g elements in group-effectiveness seem to yield to a predominance of s elements. "Level" functions give way to "field" aptitudes: the relating of the general capacities of the group to the larger problem gives way to the relating of personal capacities and skills to the *ad hoc* problems as they arise.

In the actual observation of level of functioning in a group one notes that some men have the right plans but cannot organise them into their details: others are not fertile in plans but quick to recognise the useful ones and how to organise them. Others excel in practical improvisation on the job. At each level of functional ability, there are some who can "sell" their plans, methods of organising or practical techniques and others who cannot. One man with something to contribute cannot get it over: another will find it easy to foist useless ideas, plans and techniques—at any rate for a time—on the group.

STABILITY

Stability a Normalising Function

"Stability" is not a very dynamic term for what is essentially a dynamic concept i.e. the active and continuous capacity not only to resist the deteriorating effects of stress but also to return to normal when these have passed off. To indicate an actively normalising function rather than a passively resisting inertia, "morale" might have been a better word: had one not found it convenient to use it in a more limited sense in Chapter XIV as a component of stability. "Mental stamina" might do.

The Impasse as a Test of Stability

A touchstone of character is how one copes with frustration: and successful adjustment to living is largely the constructive direction of one's reactions to such frustration.

A crucial moment therefore in group behaviour is the impasse or moment of maximum stress: when no solution of the task is forthcoming or seems possible: when a discussion culminates in an acute clash of wills or no one can think of anything to say.

One may then note (a) *how* each reacts to frustration, (b) *who* takes the initiative in de-tensing the group.

The more stressful the task and the greater the exposure to the impasse, the more deeply will the superficial crust of façade and conscious compensations be penetrated: the deeper the strata of personality that will lie revealed.

In extreme frustration tests, groups have been set impossible tasks which they did not realise to be so. Such extreme applications of stress are best avoided by observer teams which lack the high psychological skill required to "seal-off" or disperse the after-effects: teams which possess such high skill can usually get all they need in tasks of lesser difficulty and are least disposed to use them.

It should be kept in mind that a task which makes only physical demands—rather than social or intellectual ones—can throw light only on physical stamina and not on group-effectiveness. A task which imposes *no* stress is—by definition—not a task.

Types of Stresses that Contribute to the Impasse
These may be:—

a exogenous (exercised on the group from outside),
b endogenous (exercised on the group from inside),
c intrapsychic (exercised on the individual from within).

Among the exogenous stresses are: the difficulty of the task, the time element, the scrutiny and critical attitude of the observer team etc. On the whole, the group tends to close its ranks to resist such stresses: their tendency is to bind rather than disrupt it and to encourage collective effort. If they are extreme—as in the insoluble task not known to be so—they will of course eventually disrupt.

Demands from within the group will disrupt a group where demands from without may unify it. A severe test are the endogenous stresses created by group-disruptive members or tendencies: or by demands on the group made by the helpless "stooges" and "isolates".

There are other stresses which act selectively on individual members. They may be in reaction to exogenous or endogenous stresses but the major stress is their specific intrapsychic concomitant. The commonest intrapsychic stress is of course the conflict between desire to shine and desire to meet the group's demands.

"Time-anxiety" is another intrapsychic stress. In some, their fretful restless hurrying tempo indicates not so much an objective and proportionate "sense of urgency"—for which it may be mistaken—as the relentless energy-squandering demands of the self-driving compulsive-obsessional neurotic.

Some are "allergic" to strongly dominant individuals to whom they react as to the unsympathetic father figure, with either resentment or acute anxiety. Psychiatric interview will confirm that they are essentially aggressive or submissive rebels: and that relations with superiors or elders will constitute the greatest threat to their stability.

One man will work and plan happily under a stronger leader or in a small sub-clique of equals: but given chief authority and responsibility he shows extreme and incapacitating anxiety. There is evidence (one's own unpublished investigations tend to confirm it) that more men break down from the chronic stresses of responsibility and authority over others than from physical danger or deprivation. This is specifically tested for in the "Command Situations" where the candidate is given a group task, put in charge of the group and so vested with authority over it.

One of the dynamic attributes of stability (to use the Irishism) is the ability to meet phasic changes in stress: not only its increase up to extreme frustration but also its rapid lowering. An "Indolence Test" has been suggested in which one notes the candidate's behaviour with the sudden de-tension when a task is ended or "sealed": or in an interval between tests when there seems nothing for him to do. In such moments of indolence or sudden relief, the group-disruptive or anxious will often reveal themselves. The heady draught of success or sudden relief can be as revealing as the bitter draught of failure and frustration. Where the more stable can relax between efforts though ready to "go all out" when required, others will remain tense or reveal the need of de-tensing techniques like facetiousness, horse-play etc.; which may be aggressive or favour-seeking.

Enforced muscular inactivity—as required for instance in some indoor tasks—is a stress that many cannot tolerate: notably the overactive man of restless drive in whom action is an escape and muscular restlessness a manifestation of anxiety. The psychiatrist will often recognise in him the type—often of lower intelligence level—prone to hypomanic or hysterical reactions under stress.

On the whole, exogenous stresses compel the group to function as a group and so help to bind it and to distribute the stress of the task equally over its members: endogenous stresses tend to disrupt the group: intrapsychic stresses affect individual members specifically: all three put to the test the group-effectiveness of every member—especially during the impasse.

Frustration Reactions to the Impasse as a Pointer

At the very moment of the impasse, the candidate's specific reaction to its frustration should provide important, possibly critical, information to the skilled observer about his stability.

The good member of the group is well aware of his anxiety and will not hesitate to admit it to himself. It is eased to some extent by his empathic concern for the anxiety of the others which provides the incentive to de-tense the group so that they may carry on. He may deliberately retain some degree of tension if he feels it can be used as a deliberate goad or stimulus. With the disruptive or aggressive he will use tact; with the inhibited, shy or nervous, encouragement or positive suggestion. If he uses humour he will use it constructively and purposefully to de-tense the group, individual members or himself: not in self-defensive facetiousness or aggressive wit directed against others.

To the good member, frustration is the stimulus which almost automatically causes him to "collect" himself: like the attacked judo wrestler, he may have to go where he is pushed but he knows where he goes and has not lost mastery of the event. His ability to de-tense himself and the group in that impact with stress is an insurance of its emotional support and a safeguard to his stability.

Among the less adequate reactions to the impasse are the following: the frankly anxious who react with aimless and restless activity, fidgety mannerisms, a tense expression, nervous facetiousness, automatic and unintended truculence etc: the "compensators" who thrust, bluff, boast, exhibitionistically seek the spotlight or in some similar way seek to mask their insecurity: the depressives who apologise, seem mortified and blame themselves for everything; the "projectives" or "blimps" who paranoidally blame the materials, the nature of the task, other members— anything but themselves: the hysterics who express their insecurity in irrelevant acrobatics or pressure of speech which contribute nothing to the task.

Attitude to the Group as a Pointer

At the very moment of the impasse, the candidate's genuine social attitudes should stand revealed: any cloak of dissimulated consideration for others will drop to reveal the true degree of his group-cohesiveness.

A man's group-cohesiveness will on the one hand determine his effective level by helping to implement his abilities: on the other hand it will increase his stability by gaining him the emotional support of the group.

In so far as he is Group-cohesive and helps to bind the group in friendly participation, he wins a measure of appreciation and approval: his anxieties are diluted in theirs and he shares their satis-factions as well as their pains. Having solved the conflict between self-interest and the group's interests, there is less detraction from his energies, less call on his reserves: his social behaviour will be more spontaneous, natural and without *arrière-pensée:* his group-cohesiveness will lead to an inner self-cohesion which is the basis of his stability in that group.

The Group-disruptive—at greater cost of energy—derives less support from the group who may reject him. His self-driving and self-compulsion—in the effort to win its approval or compel its cooperation—makes further inroads on his energy reserves and leads to the vicious circle of self-compulsion, driving rather than leading the group, ultimate self-disruption and instability.

Such ability as has the Group-dependant or the Isolate is short-circuited by his social deficiences. He condemns himself—unless he can live a parasitic life—to live either as a compulsive neurotic driving helplessly and aimlessly, without pivot or fulcrum, in a social vacuum; or in a schizoid phantasy world of his own. He cannot hope to be a stable member of society. To the psycho-therapist he is a challenge: especially if—as often—his intelligence, "values" and ultimate aspirations are of the highest and should not be wasted to the community.

Stability is Relative to the Imposed Task

A man's stability is relative to what is demanded of him or what he demands of himself: to the field, the level, the tempo, the duration of the task. He may be stable in one field or on one level and unstable or neurotic in another. In the military field, a high stability and consistent performance is especially required of the officer. He must not only plan, organise and handle men on a sufficiently high level but also be capable of maintaining that level for long periods at high tempo under continuous stress. The man who can put up a brilliant high-level performance for a shorter period provided the stress is limited cannot ordinarily be used: at any rate in a zone of combat.

There are of course fields where he might be of outstanding value to society. It may well be true of certain fields that highest effectiveness can only be purchased at the cost of stability. If so, it may be folly not to use certain men on their highest level; but if society's profit means endangering the individual's stability, it is only fair—as well as expedient—to safeguard that stability and to spare—or even coddle—the man.

One man—out of a wartime sense of duty, unusual ambition or conscious intent to live dangerously but more usefully—may elect to function on a level above his optimum. Another—with less courage, less ambition, less interest in his community—may elect to live safely and stably at a level well below his optimum.

A man's optimum level, optimum stability and greatest value to the community may not necessarily or always correspond. But again, it seems fair and reasonable and expedient that the community should note these opted levels in their social planning and their awarding of prestige values and social approbation.

Again it may be expedient—in communal emergency such as war—to use a man where he is most needed rather than where he is most efficient or stable. The major poet might conceivably have to fight in the front line. But it must be a grave crisis indeed to justify expending the rarest abilities to meet short-term needs. I am not of course considering the inner necessity which might compel the artist to seek this experience, even if he were not particularly useful in it.

These five preliminary chapters may at this stage seem academic. There is no greater corrective to generalising nor antidote to static dogma than to watch a few hundred experimental Leaderless Groups. They constitute a psychological laboratory in the field where it is possible at every stage to test, check and counter-check one's hypotheses and clinical conclusions: an experimental "micro-community" in which interpersonal relationships and social situations in infinite variety may be continuously and precisely observed in tasks of every kind, under every degree and kind of stress.

In Part II of this book are discussed the techniques which permitted the observations on which these tentative chapters are based.

PART II: TECHNIQUES

CHAPTER VI

GENERAL PLAN OF 3-PHASE WOSB TESTING

THE WOSB OBSERVER TEAM

The constitution of the Board was three-fold and consisted of:—

a The President (Colonel) and Deputy-president (Lieut-Colonel) who up to the end of 1945 interviewed all the candidates between them: subsequently the President's function became largely judicial: the Deputy-president and Senior PSO were then constituted as "Team-leaders" and shared the interviewing:
b 4 PSO's (a Major and 3 Captains):
c the Psychological Department consisting of a Psychiatrist in charge, a Psychological Officer and 3 or 4 Serjeant-testers.

The PSO's were specialists in the "job-analysis" side of the work. As fighting officers, they had exercised the roles required of an officer both in the training depot and under the stress of combat. They were required to consider each candidate in terms of his capacity to fulfil these specific roles: and to estimate whether his functional level and group-cohesiveness were sufficient to enable him, after suitable training, to do so.

The Team-leaders and President had in addition a deeper knowledge of the military background in peace and war: they were in a position to consider (a) the genuineness of the candidate's self-identification with the military field, (b) his compatibility with that field and the likelihood that he would fit in happily.

All the information obtained by the Psychological Department was pooled so that the psychiatrist could advise the Board about:—

a the candidate's present physical and mental health:
b his likely physical and mental stability on officership level in a specific Arm:

    c his present social and emotional maturity and its likely development in the near future (specifically during training and early commissioned service):

    d points indicating special temperamental or vocational suitability or unsuitability for specific Arms of the service.

The psychiatrist interviewed a cross-section of the candidates, as time permitted. On certain types of board, he and the Psychological Officer interviewed all the candidates between them.

THE 3-PHASE TECHNIQUE

The technique here described is a 3-phase one i.e. candidates were observed in group tests before and after the interviews. Three members of the board (one from each department) constituted an Observer Team who observed the effectiveness of candidates in group tests in the first and third phases. In the second phase, each observer functioned in his specialist role: the PSO carried out the "PSO Battery" of tests: the Team-leaders and psychiatrist (and occasionally technical members of the board) interviewed: the President in his judicial capacity had a nominal 5-minute interview with each for purposes of check-up and recognition. Each observer combined general observation with specialist investigation in such a way as to enhance the value of both.

Phase 3 was optional until a very late stage in WOSB development. It became routine procedure from an early stage at several boards and was an integral part of an optimum procedure worked out at 10 WOSB and further developed at 5 WOSB. As one considers it a basic element in effective group testing—for reasons discussed throughout this book—it is the procedure here described.

Preliminary Paper Screening

After an "unbuttoning" address by the President, the afternoon of D1 (Day One) was spent in a $4\frac{3}{4}$ hour session of written work i.e. intelligence tests, health and vocational questionnaires and "projection" tests. About halfway through—when the Health Questionnaire was introduced—the psychiatrist gave a short informal chat in which he sought to allay any anxieties that the psychological aspects of board procedure might arouse.

The written material was contained in a dossier for the use of

the psychiatrist. Its analysis and summary by a Serjeant-tester
constituted a Personality Pointer to help him decide priorities in
interview and to draw his attention to matters that should be
investigated in the course of the interview. Some of the biographical details were abstracted to provide a Background
Summary for the use of the other observers on their Final Board
Proforma and also a Worksheet to be carried for reference during
the testing procedure.

PHASE I

On the morning of D2, candidates were squadded in groups
of 8: each was given a number (1 to 8, 11 to 18, 21 to 28, etc.)
and an armband or—better still—a chestband bearing his
number on front and back. In the subsequent $2\frac{1}{2}$ days of testing,
he was known and addressed by this number alone. This was
intended as a democratic gesture to safeguard against possible
nepotism: its most valuable function was to identify any candidate
at any time so that transient observations could be swiftly and
accurately noted without strain on the memory.

Phase 1 lasted about $2\frac{1}{4}$ hours (it was known as the Basic
Series) and comprised:—

a a 60-minute Undirected Group Discussion (a leaderless
  group in which candidates might discuss any topics they
  pleased in any order):

b a 40-minute Progressive Group Task (a leaderless group of
  a practical outdoor nature in which the group might be
  required to carry a heavy object over 1–3 obstacles of
  progressive difficulty):

c a 25-minute Intra-group Race (found at 5 WOSB to
  improve the value of the Basic Series out of all proportion
  to the time spent on it): the Group was selectively divided
  into two sub-groups of 4 (the "heads" and "tails" in the
  one, the doubtful "middles" in the other): these were
  raced against each other over two parallel short fast-
  tempo obstacle courses and observation was mainly
  focused on the query group. This enabled one to complete with greater precision one's ranking of the entire
  group in terms of group-effectiveness.

The object of Phase 1 was to get a balanced sample of the
candidate's group-effectiveness in the context of his group.

Part (a) aimed to project his capacity to deal with people, ideas and words: part (b) and (c) aimed to project his capacity to deal with people, material things and practical activities. Together they should provide the balanced sample one hoped to project.

The Query Conference or First Interphase Screen

The Basic Series ended, the observer team met for 10 minutes informal conference.

The aim was to pool all impressions and queries, to note discrepancies in opinion or matters of common doubt, to make manifest any individual tendencies towards "halo" or "horn" (prejudice *for* or *against*). The Query Conference should result in:—

a a provisional team estimate of each candidate's level of group-effectiveness:

b a team list of queries or doubts about the candidate for referral to specific tests or interviews in phase 2.

To get the right answers you must put the right questions. The Query Conference aims to formulate as clearly as possible the right questions arising from phase 1 and the paper screening, so that these may be put to the procedures in phase 2 best calculated to give the right answer.

By narrowing the field of enquiry and by focusing the full and specialised attention of the team on it, the Query Conference acts as an interphase sieve, filter or screen.

PHASE 2

This lasted through the afternoon of D2 and all of D3 and comprised:—

a a "PSO Battery" of individual—as opposed to leaderless group—tasks:

b the military, psychological and technical interviews.

The observer team now split up into its individual members who as specialists proceeded to investigate specific points about the candidate in order to resolve the queries raised and to confirm or rebut the general impression formed at the Query Conference.

The PSO Battery is a group of tests which aims at differentiating group-effectiveness into some of its more important component roles such as:—

a organising a group over which the candidate is put in charge (Command Situations):

b giving a talk (Interests Session):

c dealing with the human factor (Human Problems Session):

d planning a complicated project and handling it in the committee stage (Planning Project):

e the sensible use of one's physical abilities (Selective Obstacles):

f ability and interest in a special or technical field (Apparatus Session), etc.

It aims at making an estimate as to how he may be expected to function in these roles after suitable training; and especially in those roles where his capacity has been queried.

The Interim Grading or Second Interphase Screen

Just as the Query Conference pools the estimates and queries of phase 1 and acts as an interphase screen between it and phase 2, so the Interim Grading—by pooling the provisional gradings of phase 2 and revealing discrepancies of opinion and residual doubts—acts as an interphase screen between phases 2 and 3.

This extremely useful screening device—initiated at 5 WOSB in 1945—was merely a slip of paper with 3 parallel columns in which each observer entered his provisional grading of each candidate at the end of phase 2.

Immediately before the Final Exercise of Phase 3, any major discrepancies in grading were noted and informally discussed: generally there were one or two in each group. The observer team was then in a position to focus attention in phase 3 on the one or two query candidates and on the one or two queries about each. Observation sharpened in this way and focused on an ever-dwindling area of enquiry made for preciser judgment. It was preferable to resolve discrepant opinions by additional selective observation in the field—where they could be resolved—than by verbal debate and argument at the Final Board: presented too late to permit of checking by test or experiment.

PHASE 3: THE FINAL EXERCISE

Held on the morning of D4, this usually consisted of a 45-minute practical task of the leaderless group type.

The 3 or 4 groups in the batch worked on parallel obstacle courses converging on a common or similar goal. The incentive was inter-group rivalry rather than the time bogey and for this the common goal was the greater stimulus. A higher degree of stress than in the Basic Series might be imposed and would compel a response of some kind from all.

The observer team was now in a position to concentrate on one or two points about one or two candidates. In this way the Final Exercise resolves the residual queries from phase 2 and confirms—or if necessary rebuts—its provisional gradings of the other candidates.

The Sociometric Test and Screen

Now that the testing procedure is coming to an end, candidates are asked to give an indication of their capacity for objectivity and soundness of judgment by ranking the other members of the group with whom they have cooperated in difficult tasks for several days in order from 1 to 7 in terms of:—

a their ability to influence others as leader:
b their ability to be accepted and liked by others as a friend or pal.

It is pointed out that the observer team has already made its judgments and the only way of evaluating the candidate's judgment is by comparing it with that of the team.

From these individual rankings, a group ranking is calculated. Interpreted skilfully—as indeed it must be if it is not to mislead—this test can be a useful index of each candidate's dominance and acceptibility *in that group*. Discrepancies between the group's ranking and the observer team's opinion or rating should be resolved if possible: in this respect, the test provides an additional screening effect between the Final Exercise and the Final Board.

THE FINAL BOARD

On the afternoon of D4, the candidates were called in one by one before the assembled board for recognition. After their dismissal they were discussed. From the end of 1945, a psychological profile of 17 items was used for this purpose: and the candidate was rated on each item in terms of a 5-point rating.

The Final Board profile constituted a major and important advance in WOSB technique for reasons that will be discussed later. It did not aim at covering the whole field of personality but it made sure that a sufficient variety of fields were considered:

and it effectively prevented any tendency to an impressionistic dichotomy of Pass or Fail.

After completion of the profile by the board, individual reports were read to complete the picture. After discussion, the President crystallised and implemented the collective decision of the Board.

THE PSYCHOLOGY OF 3-PHASE TESTING

If reasonably well carried out, the 3-phase procedure gives one so great a sense of finality and certitude that it may be worth enquiring into its psychological justification in relation to the judgement process. This section is theoretical and tentative: but being based on introspections on the judgement process over a period of three years, during which one was required to make frequent and complex judgements, these tentative formulations may be of some provocative value to the academic psychologist as well as to the more pragmatic observer who is required to make judgements on the results of his observations.

According to older Associationist psychology, perceptive thinking is the building up from a collection of associated impressions or atoms of thought of an integrated whole. One now believes the reverse. In terms of Gestalt psychology, perceptive thinking is a progressive differentiation of a Gestalt or pattern: one perceives a new thing or idea as a whole, and proceeds to differentiate it into its component parts. To take a simple example, as one enters a room one gets a simple general impression of the room: as one gets to know it intimately, one becomes increasingly more aware of its details. The total pattern is progressively differentiated into its component parts: one proceeds from the whole to its parts, not *vice-versa*. According to the biologists, this progressive differentiation is characteristic of both the ontogenetic and phylogenetic development of awareness and response in all living organisms.

A similar process is encouraged in the 3-phase procedure. Phase 1 gives a general impression of a candidate's group-effectiveness: Phase 2 differentiates this into its component parts i.e. into such roles as planning, persuading, instructing, etc: Phase 3 returns one to the general impression. The Gestalt or total pattern has been differentiated and is now re-integrated again.

The Final Board repeats this psychological rhythm of differentiation followed by a re-integration—but on a smaller scale:

moreover, whereas the emphasis in the 3-phase procedure is on the differentiation, in the Final Board it is on the re-integration. By means of the psychological profile, each candidate is split up into his component parts or fields (actually 17 of them): one then puts Humpty Dumpty together again and the Gestalt is re-integrated for the last time.

Be it noted that from Phase 1 to Phase 2, one swings from the total field to a "close-up" or "pin-pointing" of the "query area". This implies—in WOSB technique—a *selective* differentiation i.e. one concentrates on that part of the differentiated field which is least clear and which seems of critical importance in clarifying the total picture. In effect, one explores in special detail and in greater depth those parts of the personality that suggest some possibility of failure to adjust on officer level. Obviously the more explicitly that area in the field is sought in Phase 2, the greater the likelihood of clarifying the total picture. In short, to get the right answer, one must ask the right question.

This purposeful and selective differentiation of the total field of observation links up with another principle that may be of importance. Perceptive thinking is probably more than a mere process of progressive and selective differentiation. With increasing differentiation, there seems to be a continuous referral back from part to whole; a reciprocal "field" relationship between part and whole; an oscillation of attention between the Gestalt and its component parts. Progressive differentiation and re-integration alternate and polarise each other in an oscillatory rhythm. In "field" theory, causality—as between the Gestalt and its component parts—is not so much a chain or sequence of events, temporal or spatial, as a circular and reciprocal relationship.

It would seem that only by referring and relating each newly perceived detail to the whole, can one hope effectively to differentiate that whole. The differentiation and re-integration of a Gestalt are seen to be simultaneous and reciprocal processes that develop *pari passu*. It is possibly this phasic alternation, this oscillation between the total field of observation and its parts that constitutes effective perception: and it seems to be favoured by the general rhythm of the 3-phase procedure i.e. from the general impression to the particular, then back to the general.

Somewhat analogous with this oscillation between the Gestalt or "field" and its parts is the scientific discipline employed when one refers from a general principle that is being formulated to particular instances that may test that principle: or when one refers from particular instances or processes back to their general principle. This reciprocal checking of the general with the particular ensures a logical and organic extension and growth of knowledge. But of course the relationship of whole to part is not the same as that of universal to particular, and the comparison is by analogy.

Four concomitants of this alternation of phases between whole and part may be lightly touched on because they seem of practical importance.

First is the matter of "psychological distance". In Phase 1 one gets a general view as if from a distance. In Phase 2, one approaches to get a "close-up" view of the "query area" one is attempting to "pin-point". From the "detachment" of watching the leaderless group, one switches to the "attachment" or intimacy of a more personal contact (most marked in the psychiatric interview—least so in the PSO Battery, but occurring to some extent in all the test procedures of Phase 2). In Phase 3, one returns again to the distant view and its greater detachment.

This change in "psychological distance"—this contrasting of "near" and "far"—seems to correct any falsification of perspective by over-emphasis of the "close-up" view. What looms large in the "close-up" of Phase 2 will resume its rightful size and significance in Phase 3. This phasic alternation in "psychological distance" should on the whole tend to eliminate such errors of judgement as are due to a faulty perspective.

A second aspect worth considering is the degree of activity or passivity in the mind of the judge. In Phase 1, the mind is comparatively passive as one allows the general picture to impinge on it. In Phase 2, the mind functions actively in its specialist role which now explores in depth rather than in extensity or area. In Phase 3, the intensity and concentration of the second phase relax into a more passive perception of the general and total picture. At the actual Final Board, the judgement process becomes active once more, especially in the resolving of discrepant profile ratings: there is however no uneconomic tension here as most of the active work has been done in the second phase. The judging mind may be compared to the perceiving eye which contracts its lens muscles to perceive near objects but relaxes them to see what is distant. This phasic alternation of muscular activity and relaxation prevents fatigue in the eye; and a similar alternation of active and passive perception should tend to prevent fatigue of the judging mind. Fatigue is a very real problem for those who have to make many and frequent judgements. As older men are the best judges of men—or rather, as good judges improve with age—this is of particular importance to them.

A third aspect is the phasic alternation of exploration in extensity with exploration in depth: in Phases 1 and 3 the exploration is more superficial and extended, in Phase 2 it is deeper and focussed on smaller areas.

A fourth aspect is the phasic alternation of team work with individual work: in Phases 1 and 3, the team observes collectively and together; in Phase 2, they work separately and individually. Three results of this co-ordination of shared with individual effort are:—

 a the elimination of "halo" or "horn" (prejudice *for* or *against* an individual),
 b a more effective exploration in depth,
 c a more natural fusion of specialist investigation with general observation.

It is obvious that the effect of the team—in Phases 1 and 3—will be to cut out individual "halo" and "horn". Phase 2 enables the individual observer to make an observation in depth which is all the more effective because the appropriate areas where one might begin to "dig" have been more precisely delimited in the Query Conference. There is also the isolation of the candidate from the rest of his group to assist in this temporary concentration of the field. The marriage of specialist with general observation should be most apparent (1) at the Query Conference where psychiatrist, PSO and team-leader first indicate their specialist impressions, doubts and queries for consideration by all: (2) at the Final Board where each evaluates all the pooled data in the light of his own special viewpoint.

CHAPTER VII

THE RECEPTION OF CANDIDATES

It is important that candidates on arrival should be "unbuttoned" gradually into the "selection" atmosphere: the "training" atmosphere of the military unit must be completely banished. The object of the country house is, of course, to facilitate this "selection" atmosphere in those who are being conditioned to behave regimentally in barracks. If suitably inducted and de-tensed at this stage, both candidates and observers will enjoy the proceedings and the board's work will be correspondingly easier and better.

The President's welcoming address sets the tone of the whole board. In so far as he can symbolise in his attitude the benign father—firm but kind—he will help to make selection procedure easier, pleasanter and more effective.

The distinction between "training" and "selection" must be kept continuously in mind. The psychiatrist must make an emotional adjustment from the attitude of the therapist whose instinct is to help, to that of the selector whose function is to evaluate objectively. Regimental officers—fresh from the training unit—find it particularly difficult to forego the gingering-up attitude of the camp with its urge to stimulate, pep-up and drill; to reproach men for slackness and incite them to greater efforts. Where one's object is to see a man as he is, to encourage complete spontaneity rather than to improve or train him, the most effective way of nullifying this aim is to infect the procedure with this desire to raise the tone and level by every regimental device and ritual. A President or board member who cannot learn to distinguish clearly between the "selection" and "training" atmospheres cannot hope to be suitably employed on a selection board.

In an earlier procedure, the President welcomed the candidates in the presence of the other members of the board. A less formal, more gradual, more functional procedure was worked out at 10 WOSB. Instead of the candidate meeting all the members of the board at one fell swoop—an emotional experience which he might have difficulty in assimilating—it was considered psychologically sounder for him to meet each board member on

49

his own ground i.e. when he makes his first impact with the
particular function or department of that member.

On arrival, candidates were met by the Serjeant-major—
specially briefed about his less regimental, more paternal role—
who explained the routine of the establishment i.e. meal-times,
messing, etc. He was given a number—worn on an arm band—
by which he was identified throughout the board procedure.
At the earliest opportunity, the President set the tone of the
Board in his welcoming address. Right through the initial paper-
screening, the Psychological officer who supervised it "nursed"
and de-tensed them carefully and tactfully without a formal
address. Emotionally, intelligence testing is in some ways
analogous to the testing of manhood in the adolescent rituals of
primitive societies: it induces very real anxiety which cannot be
completely removed but must be minimised.

Halfway through this screening—ostensibly to introduce the
Health Questionnaire—it was one's custom to come down and
introduce oneself in an informal chat of 7 to 8 minutes. Its
object was to allay anxieties which might arise about the psychological procedure and the psychiatric interview: and in the
course of time it embodied all the anxieties elicited in psychiatric
interviews and in the auxiliary enquiries that accompanied the
sociometric check-up (page 208).

This short address helped—so one felt—considerably

1 to make the psychiatrist's subsequent presence as an
  observer acceptable and in no way disturbing
2 to save about 15 minutes in every interview ordinarily
  spent in making preliminary contact.

After seeing him before them, it was easier for them to appear
before him: and candidates reported that any fear they might have
had of the psychiatric interview was considerably diminished.

Occasionally it has been suggested by those with little or no
knowledge of WOSB procedure, that fear of the psychiatrist
might cause a candidate to fail to do himself justice. One's
own experience is that this did not ever occur after a preliminary
de-tensing chat. The tendency was to identify the psychiatrist
with the role of doctor, and with the attitude of science and
an enlightened democracy. They regarded him, so one felt, as
being on their side. And it is probably true that any prejudice of
the psychiatrist—in so far as he failed to be completely objective—

was probably in the candidate's favour. If there were any fear—and it did not commonly exist—it was of those senior regimental officers whose interviewing skill was insufficient to antidote the inhibiting effect of red tabs.

Next morning, a few minutes before the beginning of the non-written tests, each PSO introduced himself to his group. Candidates were thus helped at the moment of making the plunge into a new phase of testing. This progressive induction by President, Psychological Officer, Psychiatrist and PSO where the candidate entered that board-member's sphere of influence seemed natural and logical and proved psychologically effective. To meet all the members at one fell swoop was more than they could assimilate emotionally: piecemeal, it was easier.

In talks to candidates, it was generally considered wise to avoid negative suggestions i.e. that secret microphones or other spying devices were not used to observe their behaviour etc. Putting a negative or a positive sign in front of a suggestion does not really alter its emotional effect: that is a very elementary axiom in practical psychology. One could however remind them in a more positive manner that while they were continuously and carefully observed during the testing time, their manners and behaviour outside that time did not concern the board: though they were requested—as a matter of general convenience—to respect the general amenities of the mess.

Over and over again one realised how considerable was the difference between the effects of a good and a bad induction technique on the ease, naturalness and efficiency of a board. With a poor induction, boards remained "sticky" and hardly seemed to warm up: with a good induction even their initial spontaneity and happy naturalness was greater than a poor induction ever managed to achieve at any time. The effect too on Army morale, on the goodwill towards officer selection and on candidates who failed to make the grade must have been very considerable.

CHAPTER VIII

PSYCHOLOGICAL SCREENING BY WRITTEN TESTS: THE PROJECTION BATTERY: THE PERSONALITY POINTER

HOW THE WRITTEN SESSION IS CONDUCTED

After the President's "unbuttoning" address, the first afternoon's session of about 4¾ hours was spent in written work. The candidate, while fresh, was given a battery of three 20-minute intelligence tests: then allowed to de-tense while entering factual data into two questionnaires: one dealing with schooling, jobs, games, social activities, army activities etc: the other with health and home background. The psychiatrist prefaced the second questionnaire with a short informal chat explaining the psychological aspects of the Board. Last of all—when suitably de-tensed, relaxed, cajoled and warmed into some degree of spontaneity—he was given a battery of projection tests i.e. Interests Questionnaire, Self-description, Word Association Test and Thematic Apperception Test: its object was to provide clues to his emotional attitudes and temperamental make-up.

The written material may be divided into three elements:—

1 intelligence tests and Educational Standard (ES); these indicate his potential functional level:

2 biography, CO's report and health record; the first two will indicate his present achievement an d how far he has developed towards realising his potentialities; his health record may indicate how he has reacted to stress in the past:

3 the Projection Battery: expertly interpreted this will give clues to his motives, interests, anxieties, basic interpersonal attitudes and the early object-relationships to parental figures that have determined these attitudes.

HOW THE WRITTEN MATERIAL IS USED

From the written material, the Sjt-testers were officially required to prepare:—

a a Personality Pointer for the psychiatrist

b a Background Summary or Potted Biography for the other observers.

The Background Summary contained salient details from the first and second elements i.e. intelligence, ES, CO's report, biography, etc.

The Personality Pointer—as one used it—contained along with the written dossier, a full summary of the factual data, a preliminary analysis of the projective material, a provisional estimate of the candidate's level of Group-effectiveness (GE) in terms of the Spectrum Rating (page 72), any queries that might be raised about him and any special interests or experiences that might be used as topics to launch the interview or to explain his contributions to the Group Discussion. Its purpose was:—

a to screen out those who might prove to be complex or borderline as a first priority for interview;

b to summarise the dossier, make a very provisional estimate of level of GE, supply queries and topics for the interview.

A further convenient use of the material was in a foolscap "worksheet" which contained skeleton details of the 8 or 9 candidates in the group with space for observations, and which could be clipped to a millboard and carried with one from test to test. Nine or ten basic items (OIR, ES, CO's opinion, age, job, father's occupation, position in family, county, etc.) were represented in abbreviated form or numerical index. In one's own worksheet, one also included: estimated level of GE as indicated by a plus, zero or minus sign: also queries and interview topics.

For reasons explained in Chapter XIX, permission was obtained —mainly at 10 and 5 WOSB's—to bring the Sjt-testers more "into the picture" and to use them as junior psychologists. Each was allowed to observe the Basic Series and Final Exercise of the group for which he prepared Pointers: to attend the Query Conference where queries from the written material might— under the aegis of the psychiatrist—be contributed to the common pool: to participate in the other screens i.e. Interim Grading, Inter-Candidate Rating and Final Board: and to cooperate in the Human Problems Session.

This use of the Sjt-tester proved to be particularly fertile at

10 WOSB. It enabled him to coordinate and check interpretation of written material with observation in the field. This marriage of Pointer material with group-observation enabled him to amplify his Pointer and produce what was in effect a true psychological report; these one found of exceptional value not only in the interview but also at the Final Board in connection with candidates one had screened and observed but not interviewed. They made possible the fullest use both of the material and of the psychological team.

This experiment seemed more than justified by the very full psychological screening of the entire batch of candidates that it permitted, by the Sjt-tester's continuously increasing skill and psychological experience, their sustained enthusiasm, increased helpfulness to the psychiatrist and improved relations with all members of the Board.

From being "backroom" crystal-gazers, psychological tipsters and guessers, they were brought right "into the picture" where they could participate, contribute and learn.

THE FIRST SCREENING ELEMENT: POTENTIAL LEVEL

This consists of (a) intelligence level and (b) Educational Standard: together these seem to provide in the vocationally inexperienced candidate the nearest we can get to his potential level of functioning.

INTELLIGENCE LEVEL

The battery of three 20-minute intelligence tests consisted of (a) a Matrix test of designs and patterns correlating highly with Spearmans g factor of abstract reasoning, (b) a verbal test correlating highly with the verbal factor, (c) a verbal reasoning test correlating intermediately with both g and the verbal factor. This gave one a sufficiently useful approximation of intelligence level if one kept in mind the sources of fallacy.

In the first instance, under optimum conditions and with individual testing as originally intended, heredity is considered to be responsible for about 75 per cent to 80 per cent of intelligence as measured by intelligence tests. Even individual testing achieves reasonable validity in all cases only if there is a psychiatric check-up to evaluate and allow for the influence of emotional factors, anxiety, fatigue, physical discomfort, age, the presence of compulsive-obsessional trends, mental habits and "sets" etc. A group test *without* that individual check-up is of necessity two steps removed from the individual test *with* it, and is a cruder approximation to the hereditary contribution to intelligence. The non-psychological members of a selection board are especially prone—after a short preliminary period of cynical disbelief—to overestimate the significance of intelligence scores and of relatively small differences in score. It is the duty of the psychological members to correct that tendency.

By giving each test equivalent scores it was possible to compare the score in one test with that in another. A high Matrix score with a lower score in the verbal test would suggest that poor verbal ability might mask the candidate's true ability. Candidates with high verbal facility might create the impression —unless warned by the scores—of a higher intelligence than they possessed.

It was found a useful practice to submit one or two candidates in every board to individual testing: (1) partly to remind the board that group testing is only roughly approximative; (2) partly to check up on borderline candidates of lowish intelligence level; (3) mainly perhaps—at any rate in one's own practice—as an individual stress task in which a psychologically trained observer might observe a complex or problem candidate intensively under some degree of stress for an hour or more.

Despite limitations and possible fallacies, intelligence rating is the most valuable single aid to selection and one could not hope to dispense with it.

An especially valuable feature of intelligence-testing in the Army was its expression in terms of percentiles of the population (i.e. in terms of the actual frequency of each level of intelligence in the general population) rather than in absolute level of intelligence as expressed in an intelligence quotient.

Intelligence-testing at Primary Training Centres gave one a first screening. The results were expressed in six Selection Grades (termed SG's). SG 1 consisted of the top 10 per cent of the general population: SG 2 of the next 20 per cent i.e. from the 71st to the 90th percentile: SG 3 Plus of the next 20 per cent i.e. from the 51st to the 70th percentile. SG 1, SG 2, and SG 3 Plus together constituted the top 50 per cent of the population. SG 3 Minus consisted of the 31st to the 50th percentile, SG 4 of the 11th to the 30th percentile. The SG 5's were the bottom 10 per cent of the population in terms of intelligence level. These proportions varied slightly in the Army because the bottom half of the SG 5's were not employable as soldiers.

In the second screening of intelligence at WOSB, it was necessary to differentiate the higher levels more fully. Expressed in roughly approximative terms, 99 per cent of the officer population were in the top 30 per cent of the population in terms of intelligence level. The average officer was within the top 5–10 per cent.

New norms were worked out in terms of Officer Intelligence Rating (OIR). The bottom 50 per cent of the population, i.e. SG 3 Minus and downwards, was considered to be OIR 0. Going upwards, OIR 1, 2 and 3 were approximately on the SG 3 Plus level, between the 51st and 70th percentile. OIR 3— somewhere between the 60th and 70th percentile—was the lowest OIR with which a candidate could be passed for OCTU without special permission from War Office. OIR 4 and 5 were approximately on the SG 2 level i.e. between the 71st and 90th percentile: OIR's 6 to 10 were in the top 10 per cent of the population. Average officer intelligence level was found to be about OIR 6 to OIR 8. OIR 10 was the highest score in this scale: its incidence in the population might be considered very approximately as one in seven or eight hundred.

It was found that a candidate whose OIR was below the average of 6 to 8 would not cope easily with officer responsibility unless he could compensate in some way i.e. by unusual experience, drive, persistence, unusually well integrated social personality, etc. With the higher intelligences—provided there was no instability or poor social contact—there was a greater reserve of trainability and educability: even if educationally limited they could often be expected to train up to officer standard. While OIR 3 was considered minimal for a commission in a non-technical arm, a slightly higher minimum—though never imposed—was probably necessary to cope effectively in a technical arm: possibly OIR 5 or 6.

The great advantage of an intelligence rating expressed in terms of its frequency in the general population is that given a certain population, once you have established the minimal intelligence ratings for certain jobs, you can calculate the number of potential candidates available for each specific job.

EDUCATIONAL STANDARD (ES)

A simple system of indicating Educational Standard by two digits proved to be of considerable practical value. For example, 11 indicates a three years university degree on the non-scientific side: 12 indicates a degree or its equivalent on the scientific or mathematical side. 21 or 22 indicates the level of Higher School Certificate or Inter B.Sc. or Inter B.A. A terminal "2" indicates a scientific or mathematical trend: a terminal "1", a literary or humanist trend.

31 and 32 are School Certificate standard: 41 and 42 imply education—including commercial and technical education—up to the age of 16: 51 and 52 up to the age of 15: 61 up to the age of 14. No lower levels were considered at WOSB.

In one's own experience the juxtaposition of a candidate's intelligence rating and ES gives the most useful single pointer to his potential level of functioning: and constitutes an important first screening element in the Pointer material. Average officer level is about 7/31 i.e. an OIR of 7 with School Certificate level of education. With average officer intelligence between OIR 6 and 8 and average officer education 31, a candidate below average in one should be above average in the other. If below average in both intelligence and education one must demand that he have some strong compensatory element i.e. unusual experience, drive or force of character, etc. If intelligence and educational standard are both high, then—with a greater reserve of capacity—more faults and minor defects may be overlooked. For a technical arm, average officer level is nearer 8/22.

THE SECOND SCREENING ELEMENT: PAST RECORD AND ACHIEVEMENT

While a candidate's intelligence and ES indicate his potential level and what he may reasonably hope to attain, his life history indicates his actual achievement: analysis of the curve of this achievement up to date should indicate its future trend.

THE BIOGRAPHY

If recently from school, one may surmise something of his personality and character from his ES in relation to his intelligence and educational opportunities. With reasonably good opportunities i.e. a sense of security in the home, no need to depend on scholarships for his education, a good boarding-school training etc., then with an OIR of 6 to 7 he should be able to obtain School Certificate standard with only moderate and reasonable application. With an OIR of 8 to 10, less or little application may be required. With an OIR of 5, 4 or 3 the going may be hard; and with lower OIR's he may never succeed however hard he tries.

Where opportunities have been poor i.e. financial or emotional insecurity in the home, antagonism of the parents to a higher education etc., even with a higher OIR than an average of 6 to 8, the going may not be so easy and one must make allowances for the extra effort required. In the poorest circumstances, a candidate of high intelligence may have received no more than an elementary education and his educational standard may be no more than 61: that is becoming rarer now that our educational system is improving and is screening out the brighter boys for further opportunity.

Generally it will be found that the brighter candidate of limited opportunity will have taken evening classes or have self-educated himself to some extent by reading etc. From the viewpoint of officer material in wartime, the self-educated bright boy often makes better material than the less bright boy whose ES is higher but who has made a lesser effort. But it is unfortunately too true that in the effort to achieve an education, many of the brightest brains have burnt themselves out: their social personalities have remained undeveloped and immature: many have become prematurely exhausted, "shut-in," "wet", or schizoid. Obviously a system which gives a lad an education with one hand and, with the other, compels him during adolescence to adopt a mode of living which kills emotional spontaneity, *joie de vivre* and natural emotional and social development is far from satisfactory. This reflection is by the way: but it must inevitably occur to any one observing and selecting large numbers of young men for higher responsibilities.

In selecting candidates who have become apprenticed to some form of engineering for technical commissions, the Ordinary National Certificate is on 32 level and the Higher National Certificate on 22 level. For a technical commission, the latter is about average officer level. One must keep in mind that the university student with Inter B.Sc. and the schoolboy with Higher School Certificate in scientific and mathematical subjects are likely to have a wider culture and range of interests than the apprentice with his Higher National Certificate, though the latter will be the more practical man. The apprentice is often keenly aware of his limitations in this respect. Practicality is not necessarily a major qualification on officer level: nor is the workshop the best—or even a good—school for the learning of man-management. The solution seems to lie in a more balanced, more practical university training or a sandwiched alternation of university with workshop.

Where candidates have had jobs, one notes whether they have been progressive in pay, prospects or experience: and their reasons for leaving. Subsequently in interview—by asking a man how he liked the job or how useful it was to him or even how useful he was to it—it is not difficult to surmise whether he felt himself adequate, inadequate or barely adequate.

Points to note in the biography are: the sports record, the proportion of individual to team activities, the degree of participation and responsibility accepted in teams, clubs and societies, and in school, social, religious and vocational activities, etc.

THE HEALTH RECORD

The Medical Questionnaire contains items about the home background which may give useful pointers: the ages of the parents in relation to each other and when the candidate was born: homes broken by estrangement, divorce, mere geographical separation or the death of a parent: the position in the family i.e. whether the youngest, oldest or only child: the only son with several older sisters: the socio-economic status of parents and sibs (i.e. brothers and sisters): whether the candidate aims at a higher economic status than his parents and, if so, whether this is producing friction. The county from which he comes; the Glaswegian, the "Geordie" from Durham, the Welshman, the Lancastrian, the Devonian, the Lincolnshire man, etc., etc.: all these have characteristics which must be recognised and allowed for. The existence of a consistently brilliant older brother may have induced a sense of inferiority. The age at which the candidate left home may be important. Those who go to boarding schools seem to mature earlier in their social relationships; and for this reason the public school seems to provide better immediately available junior officer material than the secondary school. It may be that in the long run some secondary school candidates who mature later may achieve a higher ultimate level: if it is true, ontogenetically as well as phylogenetically, that greater development goes with later maturation. A candidate with the advantage of the public school, who is still weak and undeveloped, is a poor bet indeed.

The health record may indicate how the candidate has reacted to stress in the past. A list of symptoms including some that are partly or completely psychosomatic (i.e. physical symptoms due to emotional stress) are given and the candidate asked to tick off those to which he is prone; and to indicate whether often, occasionally or rarely. Some of these i.e. hay fever, travel illness, bilious attacks etc. are associated with a highly-strung temperament. However only the experienced medical psychologist is competent to supervise the interpretation of the health record in terms of stability.

THE CO'S REPORT

While the biography indicates the trend of a candidate's development and the stamina behind it, the CO's report is an estimate of his present behaviour in the Army. Its value depended, among other things, on the interest and judgement of the CO but mainly, on the nature of the liaison between WOSB and training unit: units which sent officers regularly to attend WOSB's supplied reports of considerably greater value. The duration of pre-WOSB observation was necessarily limited: and a man might not be given much opportunity of manifesting initiative or leadership while in the "square-bashing" stage. The report however did usually raise useful queries about a candidate's weaker points.

THE THIRD SCREENING ELEMENT: THE PROJECTION BATTERY

The third screening element—a battery of "projective" tests —is the most experimental, interesting and promising but by the same token the most difficult element to interpret and teach. As "projection" is an important concept and its techniques seem to be the germinating point of experimentation in selection on leadership level, a preliminary discussion here will deal with its most general aspects and its specific application to written tests. Its specific application to behaviour in the group is discussed in Chapters ix and x; and to speech in Chapters xiii and xiv. Chapter xvii goes on still further to project—and measure—the attitudes of groups as well as of individuals, as implicit in the choices they make and the opinions they express.

WHAT IS "PROJECTION?"

The word has two psychological uses which must be clearly distinguished: in psychotherapy and in the exploration of personality.

In psychotherapy, the projection process implies the referral or attributing of one's own repressed emotional trends to others i.e. as in the prudish spinster who discerns a sexual significance in harmless gestures; the paranoiac who reads his own aggression and hate into the attitudes of others: the conflict-ridden anxiety-neurotic who sees nothing but conflict in the community: the depressive who is convinced that the world is at last coming to its "sticky" end: and indeed in the whole tribe of prophets whose *Weltanschauung* and prognosis for the community so obviously derives from their own personal horizon.

In the exploration of personality a "projective" technique is one which aims at exteriorising (i.e. projecting as if on a screen) in spontaneous uttered, written or acted behaviour the characteristic *basic interpersonal attitudes (BIA's)*—whether group-cohesive, group-disruptive, group-dependent or isolate—of the candidate.

In brief, in psychotherapy it is a referral and attributing of one's own repressed trends to others: in psychodiagnostics, it is *an exteriorising, in elicited but spontaneous activities, of characteristic social personality and basic interpersonal attitudes.*

HOW DOES ONE "PROJECT"?

One aims to elicit the most spontaneous responses a man is capable of:—

> *a* by a lulling or de-tensing to encourage an easy natural uninhibited response (as in written projection tests, the group discussion etc.);
>
> *b* by a sudden sharp increase of stress or a very great stress which by its very suddenness or magnitude jolts or paralyses conscious control and compels a natural uninhibited characteristic response (as in the stress phases of the Stress Group Task);
>
> *c* by an alternation of (*a*) and (*b*) (as in the "Human Problems Session", the "projective psychiatric interview" etc.).

WHAT DOES ONE "PROJECT"?

In so far as such a technique is successful it should (a) project a characteristic sample of the individual's BIA's, (b) provide possible clues to the early object-relationships to parental and other figures from which these BIA's derive.

The more consciously determined projection material (i.e. Interests Questionnaire and Self-description) is likelier to throw light on the BIA's: the material which draws more on unconsciously determined elements (i.e. Word Association and Thematic Apperception Tests) is likelier to indicate the object-relationships of early life.

The Thematic Apperception Test is a direct and frontal attack on the individual's phantasies around these object-relationships: an attempt to get direct evidence of the emotional bond with the parents: to what extent it is ambivalent or mature: to what extent associated with fear (of losing the mother) or guilt (with dread of punishment by the father) etc. etc. It is for this reason that it is the very germinating tip of written projective techniques.

It is not difficult to distinguish mature objective social attitudes from those which are immature and ambivalent. In the latter there may be a dependent need of the parents and especially of the mother figure: accompanied by a hatred and resentment of them—especially of the father figure—because they cannot grant him all their love. Coexistent with resentment, there may be signs of guilt about such aggression, dread of punishment and a narcissistic anxiety due to the fear of losing love.

This ambivalent and dependent attitude to the parents will tend to deposit a nucleus or core in the personality around which will grow BIA's that are ambivalent and dependent in relation to the community and to the groups within it. It will lead to a demand for favours from the group and a resentment of any demands it may make: these are felt as threats and reacted to with counter-hostility or fear.

The healthy object-relationship—which needs and accepts both parental figures and their demands—will deposit a core of BIA's which are prepared to accept the demands of the group and are likely to lead to an adult group-cohesive attitude. On the other hand, the persistent dynamic of the ambivalent object-relationship—just as it tends to separate father and mother and so disrupt the family group on which it is overdependent—will tend to grow into an immature BIA whose tendency is to disrupt the larger group of the community in whose activities it cannot take a full share.

Whereas the mature pattern is warm and spontaneous and distributes its love and resentment spontaneously, relevantly and objectively, the immature ambivalent pattern will be "spotty", inhibited, and cold in parts, impulsive or compulsive and over-vehement in others: love and hate will be distributed capriciously, unobjectively and irrelevantly.

These are of course very general and schematic statements of two extremes in a clinical scale of adjustment.

Naturally, before one can hope to detect these trends in written material, one must have had considerable experience of the transference relationships of the consulting room and clinic: and no interpretations are safe that are not supervised continuously by someone with such experience. For the medical psychologist in WOSB, it is a fascinating experience to follow up and correlate such trends from the written work through observed activities in the experimental group to the transference relationships of the interview. These transference relationships are slighter, less vehement, more delicate and therefore more difficult to interpret in the "projective" psychiatric interview than in the ordinary therapeutic or analytic interview.

WHAT DOES EACH INDIVIDUAL TEST CONTRIBUTE TO THE PROJECTION BATTERY?

In screening written projection material, it is convenient to proceed from the more conscious material to the less, from the known to the unknown, from the core to the periphery: on the assumption that it is a more scientific procedure to master the core of available factual data before going on to intuit or make clinical "hunches" from the periphery. The order one adopted was: Interests Questionnaire (IQ), Self-description (SD), Word Association Test (WAT), Thematic Apperception Test (TAT). The last three constituted the official Projection Battery but most boards devised a short Interests Questionnaire; and it is indispensable in a Projection Battery of this kind.

The Interests Questionnaire (IQ)

The Interests Questionnaire is still in its technical infancy:

c*

much work can usefully be done to formulate questionnaires which will explore effectively and quickly a candidate's range of interests and dominant attitudes and give a preliminary picture of his intellectual, cultural and emotional development.

One's own practice was to ask the candidate—before presenting specific questions of any kind—to write on one side of a foolscap sheet a 5–10 minute essay on his favourite games, hobbies and interests; indoor and outdoor, in the order in which they appealed to him. On the second page, 2 or 3 "projective" questions were put to him which varied frequently and were often improvised for the occasion: their object was as much to keep the Psychological Department creatively alert as to try out the new. Stock examples are:—

"If you had to spend six months on a desert island with one book—apart from the Bible—what would it be?"

"If you had to spend six hours in a first class railway carriage alone with any character alive or dead, historical or fictional—language being no barrier and barring actual relatives—with whom could you pass the time most interestingly? Why? What topic would you most like to discuss and what questions would you most care to put?"

Etc., etc.

The *raison d'être* of the "projective" question—with further examples—is discussed on page 188.

After the candidate had differentiated the Gestalt of his own interest-field by listing and discussing his interests in order of preference, pages three and four were devoted to specific projective questions covering as many fields of interest as possible: his attitudes to his career, his future, the Army; "high-spots" and "low-spots" and the most anxious moments in his life; people and events that had influenced him for the better and for the worse, etc., etc.

Devising an Interests Questionnaire to systematically cover every possible field would indeed be ambitious; but it would be less difficult and of considerable practical value to list the major fields and to devise projective questions that would lead the candidate to indicate those with which he is specially identified.

Spranger has suggested 6 types of "dominant value"; the "dominant value" or leitmotif of a man's life-pattern being that which he seeks in order to obtain a sense of security in life. These are:—

1 the Theoretic or Academic type who seeks to obtain security from knowledge or truth:

2 the Aesthetic type who seeks to obtain security from the enjoyment of that which he cannot change:

3 The Religious type who seeks to obtain security by appeasing God, or his own Superego:

4 the Social type who seeks to obtain security from friendship and an emotional identification with others:

5 the Economic type who seeks to obtain security from money, bargaining, acquisition, getting, having, possessions, property, etc;

6 the Political type who seeks to obtain security from power over people, dominance, etc.

But even these wide categories do not provide a complete classification. One might add for instance—in the Anglo-Saxon world anyway and increasingly in the world generally—a Sports type. Those who seek to obtain their sense of security from play on the physical level, from the use of the body and the exercise of kinaesthetic skills: presumably there is also a social element i.e. identification with the team or display before an audience. Occasionally the interest is very vicarious and consists of mere "spectating", or listening-in to a spectator, or keeping informed about sporting activities.

And how, for instance, classify the mechanically-minded who tinker with cars, radio, model aeroplanes, etc?

Tentatively one might classify interests into four large fields:—

1 *Interest in One's Body:*
   a its use and development (muscular) i.e. as in sport and mechanical skills:
   b its gratification (sensory) i.e. as in physical pleasures, food, drink, etc.

2 *Interest in Things:*
   a natural objects, plant and animal life, the country, agriculture, gardening, etc.
   b man-made objects i.e. handicrafts, technical arts, applied science, etc. (this links up with (1*a*).

3 *Interest in People:*
   a the family motif.
   b fellowship, the community motif, social sciences and psychology, etc.

c sex.

4 *Interest in Ideas or "Values":*
in ideological, ethical or aesthetic formulations.

While there is still great scope for a preciser differentiation of the Interests Questionnaire, the short four-page questionnaire proved extremely useful. What seemed especially important— as a safeguard against missing important interests—was the principle of getting the candidate to spontaneously differentiate the Gestalt of his interests in the short essay before being prompted or submitted to suggestion of any kind. The interests he listed first were indeed likely to be his major ones.

In general one may hope to get from the Interests Questionnaire an impression:

  a of the scope, RANGE and DEPTH of the candidate's interests i.e. whether wide, average or limited; whether shallow or deep:

  b of their trend or PATTERN i.e. whether balanced, compulsive or compensatory for some real or imaginary deficiency i.e. the "shut-in" personality who seeks compensatory expression in academic distinction:

  c possibly of the candidate's "DOMINANT VALUE" in terms of the Sprangerian or other classification: it may be possible to relate this "dominant value" to the candidate's BIA's or even his early object-relationships i.e. the desire for economic or political power may relate to an aggressive primarily group-disruptive attitude, originally directed against the father figure or an envied older brother.

The "Self-description" (SD)

The candidate is asked to write two short 5-minute descriptions of himself as they might be written by (a) a good friend (b) a hostile critic. In doing so, one hopes he will project his attitude to himself and his capacity for objective self-estimate. This is often experienced by the candidate as quite a severe test and calls for particularly skilled interpretation and careful co-ordination with the rest of the battery.

The self-estimate of the mature candidate is reasonably balanced: the "friend" will mention good points, the "hostile critic" weak ones.

The attitude of the less mature, less objective candidate will

be as ambivalent to himself as it is to others: there will be too
much self-love and self-concern as well as too much self-hate and
guilt: he will over-estimate himself in some things and over-
depreciate himself in others: and will feel unduly anxious about
the former and unduly guilty about the latter.

There will be a seepage of emotion from "friend" to "critic"
or *vice versa:* the critic will attempt to excuse his weaker points:
the friend will reflect a sense of guilt. There may even be a
paradoxical reaction—a strong pointer to instability—in which
the friend attacks and depreciates while the critic excuses.

Light too may be thrown on the attitude of the Superego:
whether overstrict and compelling guilt and self-depreciation, or
lax and allowing a naïf compensatory conceit.

The Self-description may suggest that the candidate is:—

a reasonably mature and objective
b ambivalent to the self, with
    1 alternately excessive self-criticism and self-conceit;
    2 predominantly excessive self-appreciation with narcis-
       sistic anxiety;
    3 predominantly excessive self-depreciation with some
       guilt or depression;
c unwilling or completely unable to attempt any self-criticism
   and therefore lacking in insight and suspect of evasive
   and hysterical tendencies.

Useful queries may be provided for the psychiatric interview,
especially by the "critic": possibly also for the Query Conference,
though it may be advisable to defer consideration of the products
of self-criticism to a later stage.

The Word Association Test (WAT)

To make of this a group test, 50 words are exposed one by
one on large cards and the candidate allowed 15 seconds to
write a written response to each. The briefing is calculated to
encourage immediate spontaneous responses. Words were
included whose associations might be expected to project anxiety,
aggressive trends, identification with the Army, attitude to
home etc. Some deliberately equivocal words like "lead" and
"box"—with more than one meaning—were included.

The simplest way to interpret the Word Association Test is
to regard it as a sample conversation in which 50 stimuli are

given and the responses noted: except that here we can analyse and interpret these reactions at our leisure without actually seeing the candidate.

The FIRST point to note about any conversation or series of expressive responses is whether it is spontaneous or inhibited and to what degree. A SECOND point is to what extent it is emotionally warm and positive; or ambivalent, erratic and negative. A THIRD point is the presence of any unpleasant emotional tone; any tincture of anxiety, aggression, guilt or anxious striving to over-compensate for a sense of inferiority. FOURTHLY one may note indications of specific identifications with the Army, civilian life as opposed to the Army, the home; specific activities, interests and people, etc.

The good candidate is generally spontaneous, natural, un-inhibited, frank, positive, and has one or more active interests. The poor candidate is likely to be inhibited or "sticky", has many blank or one-word responses (there is evidence that upward of 10 blanks constitutes a strong pointer to instability of some kind): he is likelier to reveal ambivalent trends of love and hate, dependency and resentment: to indicate a general sense of in-security, more antipathies or fears than enthusiasms, little or no identification with the field for which he is being selected.

The Thematic Apperception Test (TAT)

This consists of lantern slides depicting topics which are slightly horrific (necessarily) and implicit of conflict, which the candidate sees for 30 seconds: he is then asked to improvise a story about each and given 2½ minutes to write it down. To give some initial impetus to his improvisation (in addition to the pressure of time stress) it is suggested that he describe (a) what has led up to the situation depicted (b) what is actually happening (c) what is likely to be the outcome.

Seven pictures were available: some were calculated to elicit phantasy situations built round early object-relationships to the parental figures. Of these, one selected and used four. The first represented a younger man (with whom the candidate usually identified himself) and a much older woman: both pre-occupied, possibly anxious. This usually elicited phantasy situations around the son-mother relationship. The second con-tained a somewhat similar son-father situation. A third (which one termed "Jekyll and Hyde") represented two men: one prosperous—the other haggard, distressed and apparently poor. This often elicited phantasies around brother-brother relationships, competitive situations generally or some conflict between good and evil impulses. A fourth neutral "buffer" picture was used: usually between the son-mother and son-father pictures.

As a fifth stimulus, a blank slide was shown and the candidate asked to write a story on the thoughts that came to mind. This might produce either a frank identification with active fighting service or a complete escape from war and everything associated with it. Another occasional experiment with the blank slide was to direct the candidate to describe the worst or most anxious moment in his life. This might give clues to the types of situation that disconcert him or the nature of his habitual reaction to anxiety.

An idea one thought of experimenting with—but never got down to—was a picture of a young man, in front of a small group of people, whose relationship to that group is equivocal i.e. they may be either an approving or a disapproving crowd. A candidate's reactive phantasies to such a situation might project his attitudes to the group and the community: whether he felt himself one of them or an isolated object of suspicion, dislike or special admiration. The idea is presented for whatever it may suggest.

Interpreting the form and content of these stories is far too large a subject even to summarise: already copious contributions have been made to the literature.

So far as FORM is concerned, the general manner and style should give an impression of spontaneity or inhibition, warmth or ambivalence: whether there is any special loading of anxiety, aggressiveness or guilt. These are matters already discussed in the note on the WAT.

So far as CONTENT is concerned, the TAT is—as suggested above—a direct and frontal attack on the psychodynamics of the candidate's early object-relationships and on the BIA's that derive from them. If the dream is the royal road to the unconscious, the TAT—an elicited daydream—is the nearest approach to it in written screening technique. It is because of this that any new development and growth in projection technique will probably occur here: it is for the same reason that it demands skilled, experienced and sensitive interpretation. While Sjt-testers and non-medical psychologists can be trained to a high skill in its interpretation under supervision, their skill is entirely contingent on the maintenance of that support and supervision. It is not a test—so one feels strongly—that can be left unsupervised to anyone whose experience is not grounded in the confidences granted only to the psychotherapist in his role as physician. Without such continuous supervision, the quality of the interpretation will fall off very steeply indeed: and will soon become perniciously misleading. That a valuable technique is also a difficult one is of course no argument for neglecting to develop it. It is important that everyone in selection should have some appreciation of psychodynamic factors even though the medical psychologist must provide guidance in their more complex aspects. These factors are discussed very fully in Chapter XIV.

HOW TO COORDINATE AND INTERPRET THE PROJECTION BATTERY

In analysing projection material, one suggested the convenience of starting with the factual and conscious, and going on to the projective and less conscious.. If—*in synthesis*—one reverses that procedure, it may help one to envisage how adult BIA's have clustered and developed around early object-relationships.

The TAT may suggest dependence on the mother, resentment of the father, ambivalence towards both or an identification with benign father and mother figures. In complex-ridden, ambivalent or family-disruptive candidates, the WAT may show inhibition and lack of natural spontaneity: tinctured with anxiety, guilt and depression. In the maturer candidate it will show more warmth, spontaneity and frankness.

In the ambivalent, the SD may show "seepage" between "friend" and "critic": it may show excessive self-depreciation and a heightened demand from the self, or excessive self-appreciation and conceit, or a complete evasion of self-criticism. It is no good sign when the candidate can write little or nothing.

The Interests Questionnaire and biography may reveal strivings to overcompensate for inadequacy; in the achievements attempted and the level of aspiration they indicate; in the nature and balance of interests and in their dominant values. Intelligence level may reveal a deliberate attempt to live either above optimum effective level or considerably below it.

In only a percentage of candidates will the written material suggest a lessened stability: it is however extremely unlikely that those whose stability is diminished will give no written sign. It will usually provide relevant and useful pointers: and even negative findings constitute a pointer.

It is essential to interpret test results synergistically i.e. to relate every test result to every other test result and to the total pattern of testing. Just as in pharmacotherapy the effect of a mixture of, say, aspirin, phenacetin and caffein is not merely the sum of their effects, but a synergistic product of their particular combination; so, analogously, must clues from projective (*especially* projective) and other material be synergised if they are to point to the true pattern of personality.

It is on this account that one is inclined to doubt the value of premature attempts to validate single items in a projection battery. Similar doubts occur to one in connection with the frequent attempts to validate graphological pointers to personality: especially when handwriting is fragmented into its minutiae instead of being seen as a Gestalt.

Over quite a number of years, one seems to have acquired some clinical skill in deriving useful pointers and queries about emotional factors in the personality from the handwriting: especially where there seemed to be discrepancy with other clinical impressions. In WOSB practice one found it a useful additional projection pointer which required no expenditure of testing time and provided material written under conditions where conscious interference was unlikely and the expressive element in handwriting possibly enhanced.

As handwriting is an expressive movement like painting or drawing—calligraphy is an important source of Sino-Japanese painting and art generally (see Chiang Yee's "Chinese Calligraphy," ch. 9)—it might be expected to provide pointers to personality. Goethe, speaking of a letter written by Schiller, says, "the handwriting nowhere shows trace of weakness".

One can see in proper perspective the true clinical significance and value of the graphological pointer if one regards it as one unrelated constituent part of either a query or a clinical hypothesis. Only when related to other pointers does the real query or hypothesis emerge. Premature attempts to validate single items in a projection battery may be not merely ineffective but actually harmful to the extent that they discourage the acquirement of clinical skills. They may kill the clinical goose before it can lay the golden data.

THE PERSONALITY POINTER

Analysis of the 3 screening elements should result in:—

1 A provisional estimate of the candidate's likely level of Group-effectiveness after training, in relation to the officer's job.

2 The raising of possible queries about his (a) potential functional level, (b) group-cohesiveness, (c) stability.

3 The listing of possible interview topics to launch the interview: unusual interests like campanology, Zen philosophy, "trout-tickling", speleology, etc.: unusual experiences i.e. having lived abroad, been an ex-POW, served in another service, etc.: the nearer the topic to his "dominant values" the more fruitful.

If one adds these 3 resultants to a brief and critical analysis of the 3 screening elements one has what one might describe as a prototypic Personality Pointer.

RATING THE LEVEL OF GROUP-EFFECTIVENESS

Group-effectiveness may be rated in several ways.

a For the "worksheets", one found a simple 3-point rating of Plus (+), borderline or Zero (o) and Minus (−) quite adequate.

b For the evaluation of performance in actual group tasks, one found the 4-point GABI rank-rating described in Chapter x the most practical. It enabled one simultaneously to *rank* each candidate in his relative order of effectiveness in the group and to *rate* his actual or absolute level.

c For the Personality Pointers one preferred the more elaborate Spectrum Rating (Appendix A). On page 218, its use in the Final Board is suggested.

The idea of using the spectral colours as points in a scale derives from Dr. (then Major) Malcolm Millar. His original scale was modified very considerably at 5 and 10 WOSBs. Its lower end was differentiated somewhat fully to include an empirical classification of the commoner types of inadequate candidate as they kept cropping up in the experience of boards. It thus became a combination of a quantitative rating scale with a qualitative classification of its lower levels in terms of the types of inadequacy responsible for those lower levels.

It is this that made it especially useful for the Personality Pointer whose function was to screen out those who might be inadequate and to indicate where they might be so. It is for the same reason that one suggests in Chapter xviii its use at the Final Board as a means of illuminating and analysing the factors that make for adequacy and inadequacy on leadership level and of following up the rejected as well as the accepted candidates.

CHAPTER IX

GETTING THE GENERAL PATTERN OF THE CANDIDATE'S GROUP-EFFECTIVENESS: THE BASIC SERIES

The object of the first phase is to get a balanced sample of the candidate's group-effectiveness in the context of his group. In the Basic Series—lasting about 2 hours—he is observed (1) in an Undirected Group Discussion aimed to project his capacity to deal with people, ideas and words, (2) in a Progressive Group Task aimed to project his capacity to deal with people, material things and practical activities.

From this sample one hopes to bring to the Query Conference:—

a a provisional estimate of his general level of group-effectiveness,

b a list of possible queries about factors that may subtract from that level.

THE UNDIRECTED GROUP DISCUSSION (UGD)

ITS RATIONALE

The essence of the UGD is that it is undirected i.e. a leaderless group: no topic is set: the conversation is allowed to follow its own spontaneous directions: the group is left to initiate the discussion, to cope with the problems that arise, to terminate or initiate topics as they think fit.

Any attempt to direct the discussion will lose the special opportunities for projecting the natural spontaneous expression of personality that the leaderless group can provide. But the directed discussion has one or two useful points which may usefully supplement it.

What strikes one as an optimum procedure is as follows:—

1 45 minutes of completely undirected discussion:

2 an interim of 5 minutes during which the PSO actively brings in, by direct questioning on the last topic dis-

cussed, anyone who may not yet have spoken (this interim may not, indeed should not, be necessary):

3 10 minutes of directed discussion: a highly provocative topic of general interest—an emotional bomb—is tossed into the group to produce a high-tempo discussion.

The discussion should not be interrupted by observers entering or leaving: any necessary interruption of this kind should be inconspicuous.

OPTIMUM DURATION

In one's own experience, an hour is the optimum period for adequate observation and full use of the test as a leaderless group: 45 minutes is a minimum.

Even under optimum conditions, it takes about 30 minutes to relax every member of the group: another 15 minutes to get them going: it is the last quarter of an hour that reveals what one is looking for. By that time—in an adequately briefed and conducted UGD—even the slow-starters are in action.

A period of about 30 minutes is useful only as a rough "screen": anything less is more likely to mislead than help.

Although a fascinating test to observe, it does make demands on the observer; especially those conditioned to prefer physical to mental activity or unaware of its purpose and significance. There is a tendency to shorten the period for reasons which are largely rationalisations of a defective ability to understand or interpret it.

TOPOGRAPHY AND LAYOUT

There seems to be magic in the closed circle: in arranging the 8 candidates in a smallish circle; the observers sitting just outside the circle but not so far back that they cannot comfortably be seen with a slight turn of the head. Observers known to be there who cannot comfortably be seen will be felt by the group as critical or even hostile.

To arrange them in a semi-circle—the chord of which is occupied by observers—is psychologically bad. The end candidates of the semi-circle are isolated, the central candidate is spotlighted; the observer team obtrudes into the group, disrupts it and produces generally an unbalanced field in which one cannot hope to project natural and spontaneous group inter-relationships.

In the worst Group Discussion one has witnessed, the candidates were arranged in a shallow semi-circle—almost a straight line—directly facing a similar line of observers. As two observer teams were observing this group—each team observing one half of it—it meant that the candidates were left face to face with an equal or larger number (if one includes the visitors) of silent but highly critical observers taking copious notes. The spontaneity born of such a layout must be still-born: as indeed it was.

A variant of the closed circle which seems to be an improvement is what one might call the "coffee-table" technique.

They sit around a low square coffee-table, two opposite each side of the table: the result though geometrically a square is psychologically a circle. Observers may sit at the corners with their chairs slightly withdrawn or wherever they choose: one's own preference was for window-ledges and one preferred to change one's observation-point at least once during the session.

The first member of each group (his number is 1 or 11 or 21) is always placed in the same seat and the others are arranged clock-wise in the order of their numbers i.e. 1 and 2 along one side, 3 and 4, 5 and 6, 7 and 8 along the other three sides. In this way one can readily place every candidate, even from the direction of his voice alone. One knew his number without having to glance at his arm-band. Relieved of the need to continuously identify and re-identify each candidate (a formidable task when required to observe each group in each board), one could observe and take notes with a minimum of distraction or unnecessary effort.

BRIEFING

The PSO has introduced himself to his group immediately before the UGD and from that self-introduction he goes on to brief the test. The object is to encourage naturalness and spontaneity as quickly as possible: to raise the social temperature slightly and launch the group without actually initiating the discussion.

The briefing can be quite short. It is sufficient to point out that (1) one object of the discussion is to help them to get to know the other members of the group they will be working with for the next few days; (2) another object is to help the observers to learn a little more about them by seeing and hearing them; (3) they may discuss any topic in any order and there are no taboos; (4) there is no reason why they should not enjoy every minute of it. It is inadvisable to suggest that the discussion should be serious or otherwise.

Visitors—if any—should be introduced to them, and their purpose mentioned: they may be reminded that they are there primarily to observe the observers and the test, and not the candidates. That the observers are also under observation will be appreciated.

An alternative technique—which uses a slight degree of direction—is to place some object on the table (a railway ticket, photograph, cigarette-lighter, coin, golf-ball, pen, watch, stick, lump of coal, etc.) and to suggest this as a spring-board from which to dive into the discussion. As a method of semi-direction, it may influence the thread of the conversation slightly for a short time.

It does however rob one of the golden opportunity of observing how the group deals with a mild impasse: and which member is able to de-tense the group's initial awkwardness by starting the discussion. It seems a pity to deprive the observer team of what is an important function of the leaderless group. On the whole, a warm and spontaneous attitude on the part of the PSO seems more helpful in launching the group than the "object-on-the-table" technique.

HOW TO TERMINATE THE DISCUSSION

The discussion is best terminated at full swing: the impetus and warmth generated helps the group on to the next task. It is bad technique to stop it in the midst of an impasse (as the sensitive but uninformed observer is tempted to do): this not only deprives one of the opportunity of seeing how and by whom it is solved but fails to allow the group to "seal" the frustration of this test before passing on to the next.

It is probably inadvisable to discuss candidates seriously until the Basic Series is over and one has a balanced impression of both verbal and practical activities. But a few words at this stage may be helpful to work off steam after an hour's compulsory silence under some degree of stimulation, possibly provocation: it is also useful to "abreact" one's first reactions to certain candidates (see page 86).

A BRIEF NOTE ON INTERPRETATION

This is fully discussed in Chapters v, x, xiii and xiv: a few special points may be mentioned here.

The MANNER of a candidate's contribution to the discussion

is probably more important than its content in so far as it projects his interpersonal attitudes and group-cohesiveness: including the five social roles considered fully in Chapter XIII i.e. (1) empathy (the ability to sense other people's emotional attitudes), (2) the ability to encourage, (3) to be firm, (4) to be tactful (i.e. to balance firmness with encouragement), and (5) to "bring others into the picture" and help them to become identified with a problem or subject.

One notes the extent to which a candidate brings others—especially the shy and inhibited—into the discussion; de-tenses the group at moments of acute conflict or awkward pause by constructive humour, tact, etc.; shares the discussion or monopolises it: raises the level of discussion or lowers it: is predominantly constructive and increases the group's warmth, spontaneity and purposefulness or is disruptive and chilling.

So far as the CONTENT of a candidate's contribution is concerned, it may not be fair to judge him on so short a sample which may not embrace his special interests; especially so in the relatively immature. Together with the written material, the Interests Session, the Human Problems Session and the Planning Project it should however give useful clues as to his range and depth of general and special interests.

HOW TO RECORD AND EVALUATE THE DISCUSSION

Various graphic systems for recording the UGD have been tried. A common one was a circle of numbers, each representing a candidate in the position in which he sat. As each candidate spoke, a line was drawn from his number either to that of the member he addressed or—if he addressed himself to the group—to the centre of the circle. A small arrow at the end of the line indicated the direction of the conversation. Though a useful pictorial device for beginners, it became tiring after a few repetitions and seemed to require too much paper and time.

In one's first 2 or 3 years of observing, one found oneself adopting—in the full GD of 60 minutes (it was hardly worth while for a shorter period)—three recording methods simultaneously.

These kept one fully occupied during the session but added remarkably to one's powers of observation.

The first most useful technique was a simple serial recording of the candidates' numbers as they spoke. Incidentally, as groups were numbered 1 to 8, 11 to 18, 21 to 28, etc., one used only the last digit. Thus 1625761 would indicate seven "tribs" or contributions: the first by 1 (or 11 or 21), the second by 6 and the last by 1. In this way a long discussion can be indicated by a few lines of figures.

To bring significance to these lines of figures, one qualified them by a variety of signs, symbols, arrows, under-linings, over-linings, etc., etc.: coded to indicate whether the "trib" has been constructive, has raised the level of discussion, has been disruptive, humorous, addressed to a particular person, etc., etc. It is not difficult to devise a shorthand code to cover most of the possibilities and it is best to devise one's own private symbols as one's observations extend. It is amazing how much can be compressed into a square inch or two of space and how easily it may recall the course and temper of quite a long discussion.

A second technique—of lesser value—was a quantitative record of "tribs". The numbers 1 to 8 are placed under one another: as each candidate speaks, a small vertical stroke is made opposite his number: each fifth "trib" is indicated by a horizontal stroke crossing the previous four. This is of course the method used by medical students, bacteriologists, pathologists, etc., to count the bacteria or blood cells on a microscopic slide. This quantitative record of the volume of each candidate's contribution can also be computed subsequently, from the previous serial recording.

A third more intermittent record—in shorthand or abbreviated longhand—is the noting of "verbatim samples" of characteristic conversation: especially those that crystallise a man's attitude, leitmotif or life-pattern. One exploited too the mnemonic value of inventing nicknames for each candidate; and of doodling facial profiles which caricatured prominent features and noted the presence of moustache, pipe, spectacles, baldness, etc. Where one dealt with large numbers of candidates and—as psychological observer—endeavoured to screen them all, every possible aide-memoire to their recognition was appreciated.

It is of course not necessary to make elaborate records, or indeed any: but for personal record, research or differentiating one's awareness of human behaviour they are extremely useful. In evaluating personality, every psychological observer is well aware of the continuous temptation to impressionism, to letting intuition replace, rather than follow and enhance, precise observation. It is amazing how little this recording interferes with one's actual scanning and observation of the candidate: in any case one should not stare. With a standard layout in which number 1 always occupies the same seat and by adopting a relaxed position in one's own chair, it need not be obvious that one is doing anything but an occasional doodle on one's worksheet. It is the unsystematic and inexperienced observers who seem to disconcert the observed by their recurrent spasmodic scratching and their worksheets held high.

After several years of experience with these three methods, they were partly replaced by the GABI rank-rating (page 97). But every approach to a total or Gestalt appreciation must be counterbalanced, one feels, by increased attention to detail: and there seems every likelihood that many more techniques of recording spoken and acted behaviour will have to be elaborated.

THE PROGRESSIVE GROUP TASK (PGT)

ITS RATIONALE

The PGT here described consists of two parts.

In the first part—lasting about 40 minutes—the group is required to carry a heavy, unwieldy or delicate object ("Oscar") over about three obstacles of progressive difficulty: the last requiring functional planning of a definitely high order (such as practicality alone will not solve) and likely to produce some degree of necessary frustration before it can be solved. To illustrate the pattern and principles, a prototypic PGT is briefly described.

Obstacle One is a wooden wall about 10 feet high, over which the whole group with their burden must pass. The obstacle must be wide enough to give each member a chance to participate. This is an easy "wide entry" obstacle whose object is to "shake down" the candidates into a unified working group.

Obstacle Two is a stream-minefield (i.e. an area which must not be touched), etc. to be crossed either by an improvised bridge, ropes, a near-by tree, etc. A choice of material suitable for improvisation is left by the obstacle. This "narrow entry" obstacle permits of effective action on a somewhat narrower physical front than Obstacle One: with the result that it will sort out the "heads" and "tails" of the group i.e. those who initiate the solution and those who merely follow. It does tend to give a

preliminary idea of the hierarchy of power or the order of dominance and effectiveness in the group.

Obstacle Three is of the "POW barbed-wire" type i.e. the
barbed-wire is of sufficient depth and height to make it really
difficult to get the group and "Oscar" and the weaker members
of the group over (the task of course is to get *all* of them over).
This "wide-entry" obstacle provides a wide front along which
the group may deploy itself and which permits of the immediate
active participation of every member.

In the second phase of the PGT, the group is relieved of
"Oscar", divided into two sub-groups of 4 and raced over two
parallel faster miniature task-courses consisting of 2 or 3 simpler
tasks.

In ranking the group after the first phase of the PGT, one is
usually fairly definite about the "heads" and the "tails" but not
so definite about the "middles". It is these "middles" or "queries"
that one puts into one of the sub-groups: the other will contain
the "heads" and "tails" who seem definitely adequate or inadequate.   Or one may use the sub-grouping to separate a very
dominant candidate from a very immature one or from one who
is not a responsibility-seeker but may prove to be a responsibility-
accepter.   The PSO may quickly consult the opinions of the
observer team before deciding the composition of the Query sub-
group.

By concentrating one's attention on this Query sub-group,
without especially seeming to, one is in a better position to rank
the entire group for group-effectiveness: and the Intra-group
Race—as this phase might be called—seems to improve the value
of the Basic Series out of all proportion to the 20 minutes expended
on it.

By narrowing the field of observation and by the more intensive observation of that narrowed area which it permits, a very
considerable screening effect is obtained.   It breaks up the
tendency of observers to think in terms of a dichotomy of good or
bad, adequate or inadequate, "head" or "tail", pass or fail.
And it compels attention to the prime task and test of the Board
—the Query candidate.

OPTIMUM DURATION

Forty-five minutes to an hour gives the group sufficient time
to extend itself, to cope with tasks that impose some frustration

and to project or exteriorise its collective and individual levels. The Intra-group Race—as an additional 20-minute refining screen—adds considerably to its efficiency.

BRIEFING

Candidates are briefed by being taken over the course: phases one and two are briefed separately. They are told they are to take "Oscar" over the obstacles in the minimum time possible. A "bogey" time for the course may be given: a recurrent time signal (i.e. "5 minutes gone" etc.) may also be given and its pros and cons are discussed on page 91.

Courses are constructed to be as self-briefing as possible: the more automatically the layout presents the actual task the better. Objects not to be touched may be painted red if they cannot be dispensed with: paths not to be taken are roped off: shallow water may be used as a visual and wet reminder of trespass or obstacle.

"Phantasy" briefing is bad practice: one does not ask them to imagine situations or conditions which do not exist, i.e. spies, enemies, bottomless chasms, concealed traps, etc. This imposes too much strain on the memory and the imagination, lends itself to a variety of interpretations, leads ultimately to a *reductio ad absurdum* in the briefing: and does not make for standardised test conditions. It is best merely to indicate that the group is to cross certain obstacles: that an object is to be moved from here to there: that certain areas or things are not to be touched.

DESIGNING OBSTACLES AND PLANNING TASKS

In designing obstacles, it is useful to consider them in terms of Lewinian topology.

The "entry" to the obstacle is of some importance. Where it is narrow—as in bridging two walls by a shortish pole, where only one or two candidates can at any moment approach the actual initiation of the solution—only the more dominant or effective candidates can be observed easily at the critical stages of the problem. It will tend to screen out the "heads", or perhaps only the more dominant members if the group is ineffective.

A "wide entry" obstacle does allow every candidate to participate in the solution and to be seen in action all of the time: it is a safeguard for the immature, the shy and the responsibility-accepters who may be quite adequate and capable and ready to accept responsibility but will not seek it or "thrust" for it.

Useful for certain specific purposes is the "double entry" obstacle which candidates must approach from both sides i.e. bridging a gap, moving a heavy burden over a high obstacle. It can be used to divide the group into two sub-groups for any purpose i.e. to separate competing individuals, to compel others to take action, etc. It can be especially useful in the Final Exercise: one can isolate, say, two residual Query candidates who are borderline, immature, unusually inhibited or passive and put them in a position where they are compelled to reveal such capacity as they have. This putting pressure on the candidate to take action is intermediate between the leaderless group and the Command Situation where he is given authority over the group and enjoined to use it.

Of some importance too, is the "total area" of an obstacle. For example, a bridging operation to be carried out over a number of low wooden platforms will spread the group out so that every candidate is easily visible. It provides a larger peripheral circle along which observers may move freely: and permits of dilution of the observer team by a comparatively large number of visitors (sometimes necessary for teaching purposes) without appreciable chilling of the observational field.

In planning a PGT, it should of course be progressive in difficulty. The "narrow entry" obstacle is best in the middle: it does temporarily and mechanically disrupt the group somewhat and would be quite unsuitable as a first obstacle. As a third or last obstacle it might be used for a special purpose and on a special occasion. A task of exclusively "narrow entry" obstacles would bring out the worst in any group.

A useful formula for a 3-obstacle task is that described above as prototypic:

1 an easy "wide entry" obstacle to allow the formation of a working group:
2 a more difficult "narrow entry" to test the group now formed and to sift out obvious "heads" and "tails":
3 a really difficult and frustrating "wide entry" to allow every member to contribute what he can.

It is advisable to keep the pattern fluid and experimental, to have ample alternative obstacles at hand, to adapt the pattern to the type of group: and from time to time to try the effect of new, strange or unsuitable patterns.

It is more difficult to record a PGT than a UGD and eventually one expressed one's results directly in the GABI rank-rating.

One did however experiment with an attempt to record it along Lewinian and topological lines. Techniques for recording group behaviour must eventually be developed if the group is to be studied scientifically: and as the Lewinian approach seems rich in possibilities, one's own attempt will be described.

As each candidate participated in the task, his number was jotted down in relation to a series of vertical lines and to two horizontal lines (spaced about an inch apart).

The vertical lines (in clusters of 3 to 6) represented phases in an obstacle: if there were 3 obstacles there would be 3 clusters. The more difficult the obstacle, the more time it took; and consequently the greater the number of phases in it and the larger the cluster of vertical lines necessary. An easy obstacle might require 3 lines: a difficult one, 6 or more.

The horizontal lines, drawn through the verticals gave one a 3-point rating of the candidate's level of participation. If it were constructive and actively furthered the task or raised the group's morale, it was entered above the top line. If he participated willingly but without adding materially, it was entered between the two lines. Below the bottom line, it indicated a negative or disruptive contribution: the latter might be indicated by an arrow pointing to the left against the direction of the task.

At each phase in an obstacle, each candidate's contribution was indicated by entering his number to the immediate left of the vertical line representing that phase: but on a level which indicated the quality of his contribution.

The addition of various signs, symbols, arrows, etc. qualified the contribution i.e. whether co-operative, de-tensive, purely physical, etc. This 3-point rating could easily be converted into a GABI 4-point rating by picking out and circling the occasional very good candidate in the top space.

CHAPTER X

HOW TO CONDUCT, INTERPRET, EVALUATE AND REPORT THE LEADERLESS GROUP

In the ability to interpret and evaluate the Leaderless Group objectively, discriminatingly and reasonably scientifically lies the quintessence of WOSB technique.

CONDUCTING THE LEADERLESS GROUP
ATTITUDE OF THE TEAM AS A WHOLE

The aim is to create an almost neutral but slightly benign setting or field in which the varying but controlled stresses of the task will project each candidate's group-effectiveness. The observer team must keep in mind that while they are observing candidates in a group task, they are part of that field: to the extent that they are felt to be benign and friendly, the group will project itself more spontaneously: such frustrations as they meet will arise from the task and the group itself.

They should be visible to the group, yet unobtrusive and inconspicuous. Observers who gather in knots, laugh misguidedly, criticise noticeably, converse in an over-loud *sotto voice*, are too obvious and too frequent in their note-taking, too restless in their movements, or otherwise fail to efface their personalities, may be felt as unsympathetic, "superior" or even hostile. The observer who obtrudes his personality is unfair to the candidates and the PSO, and is detracting from the value of the test: consistent failure to appreciate the need for self-effacement suggests unsuitability for work in selection. Visiting observers may have to be instructed in these matters: the observation field—where men are at work—is no more a place of entertainment than the Sjt-tester's testing hall.

Observers should certainly not urge candidates to do their bit, they should merely observe how they do it: once briefed, the candidates should be unhampered and unaided and "left to it". They should refrain too from the "MCC" type of remark i.e. "well done", "hard lines", "jolly good show", etc., etc. It is intended that the group should endure its own stresses and de-tense them: it is no test of the group's powers if this is done for them and if the task is robbed of its *impasses*. This bad habit easily grows to a vice and indicates a failure to cope with the empathic frustration created in oneself by the group's efforts and strivings: this should be transmuted to an enhancement of one's intuitive understanding of the group rather than be wasted in sabotaging its task. It of course derives also very naturally from the encouragement so desirable in training but so undesirable in selection outside certain aspects of the briefing and initial reception.

If there is any "sealing-off" after frustration to be done, it is best done by the PSO alone—*after* the test is over.

However, while the principle of a benign neutrality remains, there *are* occasions (i.e. when a candidate falls into a brook, for example; or has been unusually unlucky) when common sense indicates it is perhaps kinder to laugh *with* him than adopt a somewhat unnatural impassivity which may seem hostile.

It did occasionally seem helpful to "abreact" or work off one's resentment of a flagrantly ill-mannered candidate at an early stage. One found that if one—in conference after the Group Discussion or in the Query Conference—deliberately ridiculed a candidate on whom one had fastened a "horn" (a negative halo or prejudice), one found it easier to sweeten one's attitude into subsequent objectivity. Indeed by freely and deliberately abreacting both "horns" and "halos" at this stage, one gave the candidate juster consideration in the long run.

ATTITUDE OF THE PSO BETWEEN TESTS

The PSO is the link between observer team and group: to some extent he participates in both. His role is the more difficult in that he is both observer and to some extent participant: he must be sufficiently friendly and warm and attached to the group to encourage their spontaneity without actually leading them: yet sufficiently detached to observe, interpret and evaluate their behaviour.

His attitude must therefore seem one of non-discriminating benignity: sufficiently spontaneous to put them at ease and launch them: not sufficiently positive to lead them or give them pointers to the type of behaviour he approves of or hopes to find.

He must resist the tendency—by the "on-the-double" smartness of the training depot—to create a sense of urgency which derives from himself and not from them. If his disposition is stern and grave, he must avoid letting his Superego cast a shadow over the group so that they seem more conscientious, responsible or mature than they really are. On one occasion when an over-keen PSO, as yet inexperienced, was projecting his somewhat "high-pressure" personality into the group, the author was tempted to point to a cow that had strayed up and to suggest, not to the PSO, that the perfect PSO is rather like a cow: continuously and benignly interested—but non-interfering. The PSO who is so insecure that he is compelled to obtrude and advertise his own personality is obviously not yet fitted for the objective evaluation of human beings.

The objective PSO will never particularise—without special reason—but will address the group: he will never, by word or expression, give the slightest indication of condemnation or depreciation. If he uses praise, it will be praise of the group: then, only to de-tense the group or "seal off" a task involving severe frustration. If it seems necessary—so that they may start the next task afresh—it should be done at the end of the task, never during it: and this by a few encouraging remarks to indicate they have made a fair attempt. To do so during the task is to rob it of its impasses.

A possible exception is the "dud" candidate who is severely discouraged. It is much better, of course, if the group can deal with him: if not and if it is felt that he is unlikely to reach officer level and the testing procedure may impair his confidence, one may encourage him inconspicuously. But the need seems rarely to arise. Indeed the need for "sealing off" the group seems also to be of rare occurrence. The more difficult a task, the happier does the group seem when it is over. The intensity of the frustration and of the relief when it is ended seems to produce a mild elation: and a feeling that as the task has been so difficult, they have done well to get through it somehow. An appreciative remark at this stage may help and will not prejudice the testing.

The PSO should be in full control of the test: no briefing or directions should be given the group—nor any audible comments made—except by him. It is essential that other team members, whatever their rank or seniority, should never usurp his catalytic role or make it difficult. Nor is it fair to engage him in discussion: his is a full-time job in that he must both brief and observe: if one is observing adequately, one's attention should be fully occupied. Needless to say, no directions should be given to the PSO nor any criticism of his technique made on the field when

D

candidates are present: these are properly dealt with when the board is in conference, either at the Query Conference or the Final Board.

We have here emphasised the neutral benignity of the PSO's attitudes.   Like the psychotherapist he must have sufficient strength of character to efface himself, to fade into the background and allow the candidates to project their own personalities. But it is also true that like the good psychotherapist, if he has sufficient experience and psychological flair, he may at a later stage learn to use a more active technique on occasion without loss of objectivity.

He is of course mildly active to the extent that he launches the group, raises their initial social temperature and relaxes them into spontaneity.   They should not start from cold: from the exigencies of time alone, they must be warmed up a little, at any rate not allowed to freeze: thereon after, they must be allowed to create their own warmth as part of the task.

There are occasions—in the Human Problems Session, the Interests Session, even the Leaderless Group—where an experienced PSO, under adequate psychological supervision, may take on a more active role.   Where he may purposefully interrupt or provoke the group and hold them to the stressful part of the task when they are shirking it.   Where he may break the rule of not particularising and may individualise the stress in any given test so as to increase it for one and decrease it for another (qv. Chapter xvi on the Final Exercise).

Members of a team for selecting potential junior leaders should be at least of high average officer intelligence: a matter, of course, for those who select the selectors.   If not, they may—unless their objectivity is exceptional—find difficulty with the brightest candidates, may project a lack of understanding into dislike or negative halo and may on the whole fail to do justice to the potential cream of the leadership.   Intelligence is of course not the only or most important factor in objectivity of judgement but it is sufficiently important.   Age and experience and withdrawal from the field of competition may help.   A sense of intuition, unguided by intelligence or thorough observation, is a menace though it knows well enough what it likes: the best intuitive minds will probably be the last to trust to intuition unsupported by data and observation.

One has already suggested that good judges improve with age and one finds that one cannot normally and reasonably expect long-term predictive judgements about potential leadership from anyone under 35 or thereabouts. To expect it in those under 25, however talented and wise (and one has seen selectors much younger) is perhaps too much to ask of them; and not quite fair to those who are being selected. It almost constitutes exposure to the moral temptation of a form of "power-drunkenness" to which even older men may succumb when entrusted with the power to influence the careers of others.

Up to 35, they should be acquiring the raw material of their experience. In so far as they are professional psychologists, they can serve a rich apprenticeship in the technical procedures of selection and the opportunities for observation: and may make provisional surmises and ratings under the supervision and guidance of an experienced psychologist.

Selection on aptitude level may be done by much younger men and is in itself a natural preparation. Though even here, the handling and disposal of the "complex 25 per cent" should be supervised by a medical psychologist who would ordinarily be an older man.

ATTITUDE OF THE PSO DURING TESTS

Briefly, lucidly and completely, the PSO should explain the task and the conditions under which it is to be carried out: then he should freeze immediately into a relaxed benignity. After the initial briefing—which ordinarily should require no supplementing —there should be a minimum of interference with the group.

If briefing is sufficiently lucid and complete, there will be no need for questions; and the asking of a question will often constitute a pointer to anxiety, excessive dependence, muddled thinking, limited intelligence, desire to attract attention, etc.

Needless to say, the briefing should not be followed by the usual training depot "any questions"? Commands or the tone of command are out of place: it is the candidates' leadership that is being tested: that of the PSO must be taken for granted. Groups racing each other should be briefed by one PSO and any additional briefing given by him alone.

One or two general points may be made:—

1 Briefing should be standardised into 4 or more points typed on a card: once an optimum briefing has been decided on, these

points should be rigorously kept to: the PSO may express himself in his own natural idiom but should not deviate from the standardised points.

A number of PSO's using their own individual briefings and continuously improving on them will eventually produce a set of conditions in which no two groups are being submitted to the same test. Only if tests are administered under standard conditions will it be possible to estimate and validate their reliability.

Yet with the need for a standardised core, there is also the need for growth: and—this may seem paradoxical for the moment—the need for a germinating point of deliberate improvisation in every test. In discussing the Human Problems Session (Chapter XIII), it is pointed out how this may be done by trying experimental procedures towards the end of the test on candidates who have ceased to be queries and about whom one has made up one's mind. In leadership-selection, still in its very experimental stages, one cannot progress without cultivating that germinating point of improvisation in technique. It incidentally ensures and maintains spontaneity and flexibility in the minds of the observer team.

While such improvisation will produce new ideas and techniques, any essential change in the briefing should be decided only by the Board as a collective; and not by any individual member. That is, if selection is to be scientifically validated and related to its purpose.

2 So far as possible the layout or topography of the task—this applies to practical tasks—should be self-briefing i.e. should automatically explain the task (page 82). This should incidentally eliminate the bad practice of "phantasy" briefing: where the candidate is required to imagine a set of conditions which do not actually exist and which various candidates may interpret in different ways or forget i.e. "this is a bottomless chasm", "this area is heavily contaminated with poison gas" etc.

3 Negative points are best not made. Over-explaining or anticipating points before they occur is more likely to arouse apprehension than to allay it. Part of the task is to realise in anticipation the significance of certain of its phases or sub-problems: a too detailed briefing may prevent the candidate revealing his capacity to appreciate the significant.

4 One important point is to what extent should the group be

left to create its own sense of urgency and to what extent may this be stimulated by the briefing?

By racing groups against each other, an effective time incentive is provided in (a) the second phase of the Progressive Group Task i.e. the Intra-group Race (b) the Final Exercise. Probably the best procedure ordinarily is to indicate that the task is to be done against a time factor: and either to quote "bogey" for the task or indicate that "Oscar" must be over the last obstacle within a certain time limit, or both.

A procedure that has been tried is a recurrent time-signal i.e. by calling out "15 minutes gone", "20 minutes gone", etc. This may be harmless as a mere indication of the time, if it is unaccompanied by exhortations of any kind. One's own preference, once the task is clearly briefed as urgent, is to leave the group to create its own tempo: to reveal its own sense of urgency and appreciation of the time factor—and that of its individual members—without any recurrent reminders or any stimulation of time-anxiety.

SOME NOTES ON INTERPRETATION

Some general principles broached in Chapters v and ix will be amplified in Chapters xiii and xiv in relation to the Human Problems Session and the psychiatric interview. Here we will pick out points of more immediate relevance to the observation of Leaderless Groups.

COMMENTS ON LEVEL

A source of fallacy to be kept in mind is the need to dissociate the *collective* level of the group from the *individual* levels of its members: to avoid carry-over of "halo" or "horn" from the group to the individual. This the GABI rank-rating described later in this chapter will automatically help one to do.

A team of maturely co-operating mediocrities of lowish level will sometimes carry out its task quickly and efficiently: though in a well-planned progressive task this should not be possible to its very end. Yet despite a goodish collective level, it may not contain one individual who can be trained to function on officer level.

Another team of less maturely co-operating, more individualistic but potentially bright or brilliant candidates will achieve a low collective efficiency. The homogeneous mature low-level group may be more effective than the heterogeneous immature high-level group. One must therefore consciously correct any tendency to overestimate those in the effective group and to underestimate those in the ineffective group. Group-cohesiveness is an aspect of social maturity and—provided sufficient ability for the job is there—training should assist its maturation.

One quite important point is how a man's actual or *effective level* as seen in the task compares with his *potential level* as indicated by intelligence, education, experience, etc. If there is consider-able discrepancy between what may reasonably be expected of him and his actual performance, that raises the query, what prevents him realising himself? Is it social inexperience, poor "contact", impaired morale, loss of stability, etc.?

On occasion one may usefully ask, is his *level of aspiration* unduly high or low? Is he aiming too high, possibly to compensate for some sense of inadequacy: or too low because he has been profoundly discouraged? This fringes on the medical psycholo-gist's function—with whom one can usefully cooperate in the matter—and is discussed more fully in Chapter XIV.

COMMENTS ON GROUP-COHESIVENESS

In respect of group-cohesiveness, we have already discussed three types of individual reaction (Chapter V). We may here usefully summarise—in composite—their social characteristics as projected in the leaderless group. In Chapter XIV we will consider them further in relation to the general psychodynamics of per-sonality and the particular psychological make-up of those in whom they are found.

The predominantly GROUP-COHESIVE individual is relatively more group-centred than self-centred. He attempts to bring every one into the picture: he binds the group and raises its morale, by stimulating such group-cohesive tendencies as exist in it and by counteracting and controlling those that are group-disruptive. He demands loyalty to the group and its purpose, rather than to himself: as well as some contribution to its task or morale. In return he knows how and when to convey to each member—to the extent that he needs it—the approval of the group and his acceptability to it.

He can stand stress reasonably well: partly because he is sufficiently objective to know when to fight and when to run, when to attack and when to yield: partly because he has the group with him and knows it. Under frustration, his empathy and compassion guide him so that he knows when to stimulate the group and when to de-tense it by tact, constructive humour, etc. until the difficulty has been overcome.

He plays down explicit dominance and relies rather on persuasion and collective discussion: yet manages not to sacrifice his own spontaneity but rather to enhance it. He achieves co-operation not so much by giving explicit orders as by helping to reveal and clarify the objective demands of the situation (what we later call the Law of the Total Situation or LOTS): and by indicating how each member can most usefully participate to meet those demands. He refers authority for every demand therefore to the actual situation rather than to himself: and does not so much demand participation as facilitate it.

The predominantly GROUP-DISRUPTIVE individual is relatively more self-centred than group-centred. He tends to obtrude his personality exhibitionistically into the centre of the picture, to demand personal loyalty rather than loyalty to the group, to derive authority from the individual—especially if it be himself —rather than from the demands of the situation.

In influencing the group, he prefers explicit commands and orders, often for no other reason than to dramatise his personal dominance: dominance is his ace card and he may regard a successful bluff as a high achievement.

Because of an underlying sense of insecurity for which his aggressiveness is an over-compensation, he is not objective enough to know when to fight and when to run away, when to thrust forward and when to give way. Because he thinks—or rather feels—in terms of challenge, personal prestige and competition rather than cooperation, group-binding and problem-solving, his tendency is to fight things out rather than work them out: on balance, his contribution will be progressively disruptive.

Because he *gives* less to the group—which they sooner or later perceive—he *gets* less in the way of emotional support. He must perforce drive himself and drive others: an inner compulsion makes him pit his strength and dominance against those with whom he should be cooperating. In the vicious circle of group-driving and self-compulsion, of anxiety, exhibitionism, aggression and challenge, his energy expenditure is uneconomical: and must inevitably diminish his stability and render brittle such leader-ship as he may achieve.

The GROUP-DEPENDENT and the ISOLATE either cannot or will not cooperate: either because of a schizoid barrier of morbid introversion and indifference to the group: or because of a neurotic barrier of shyness or social inhibition which makes it difficult for him to link himself with the group's effort.

The inhibited neurotic "dependent" or "isolate" reacts to group stresses by frank anxiety; or attempts to de-tense himself by nervous facetiousness, excuse-making, restlessness, self-depreciation, etc. On the other hand, the "shut-in" or schizoid "isolate" may seem apathetic and show little emotional reaction to stress or indeed to anything. Whereas the neurotic "dependent" or "isolate" will feel anxious because he *cannot* participate, the schizoid "isolate" will feel anxious because he cannot *avoid* participation.

Some of the varieties of these 3 species are interestingly illuminated in the spontaneities of WOSB slang.

Among group-disrupters are the "thrusters"; the restless "compensators" for a sense of inadequacy: the "spivoid" anti-social smart-alecks who hope by dint of toadying, exploiting others, boasting, exhibitionism, well-timed aggression or by any other means to gain credit and influence while avoiding any honest or adequate contribution to the group's purpose or welfare: who hope to trick the group and impress it at the same time. There are the strong but ruthless, difficult, anti-social personalities—possessed by a daemon of disruptiveness—for whom no particular name has been invented. In the Spectrum Rating, they rate as "Indigo A 6": they might quite simply be called "disruptives".

Among the "dependents" are: the passive rope-holders and landscape-scanners, the awkward stooges, the "passengers" who have to be carried—sometimes physically—over the obstacles, the "fringers" and back-seat critics. Among the "isolates" are the "shut-in" or "schiz" types; the "spiky", "angular", etc.

So far as level of ability is concerned, there are the occasional "zeroes" (OIR o) whose intelligence level puts them in the lower 50 per cent of the population (Army screening usually prevents their being sent to WOSB) but who are very active on their own level. There are the "monkeys" whose contribution is one of continuous athleticism but whose general level is low. The "doom-merchants" are pathetically keen, conscientious, desirous of pleasing but their level is deceptively low. Because they are "nice boys" of pleasing alert respectful manner and acceptable accent but of poor judgement they may—if not discovered early—lead men into needless danger and trouble. Yet, because of their charm, they may be carried over lesser crises to a major one where they have none but themselves to rely on. It is here that the battery of intelligence tests followed by individual testing and observation can be of special value.

Another large group are the "immatures": known in WOSB as "NY's" (NY = Not Yet). Their immaturity may be due to sheer youth and inexperience of people, or part of a general failure to develop emotionally or socially because of an inhibiting home influence. Certain types of Scot, Yorkshireman, Welshman or country lad generally (also lads who have had to overwork to obtain a good education from a poor home) tend to be social "slow-starters": as a rule, they catch up quickly, given suitable opportunities. The boarding school boy is generally more socially mature for his age than the day school boy.

COMMENTS ON STABILITY

We have already considered 3 important factors in a man's stability. Later, these are considered in detail: here we will summarise the more important clues that the leaderless group may reveal.

The first factor has already been hinted at in this chapter: the correspondence—or gap—between a man's actual or potential capacity and the level required by the job. If the gap is too great, he will be incapable: if it is almost too great (so that he must try too hard) he will be unstable. Similarly if the discrepancy between his actual ability and his level of aspiration (what he can do and what he tries to do) is too great, his stability will be diminished or lost. The lazy trouble-dodgers will of course put no strain on their stability.

We have already considered how a man's group-cohesiveness, the second factor, will stabilise him: and how his lack of it, by separating him from the group, will unstabilise him.

A third important and complex factor is the extent to which his past experiences and present health predispose him to success or failure on the level on which he should ordinarily be quite adequate i.e. his morale. If he has had consistent failure and frustration, he may be beaten before he starts and his actual capacity may never be realisable. Once the vicious circle of

D*

falling morale and lessened confidence has gathered momentum it is difficult to reverse. Apart from an analysis of his life-history by the medical psychologist in the interview, important clues and proofs of low morale will be provided by his reactions to frustration in the impasse i.e. anxiety, restlessness, boasting, etc.

The sort of questions the non-medical observer will keep in mind when considering stability—for referral, if necessary—will be:—

Has he got the ability?

Is he aiming too high or trying too hard?

Is his "contact" good enough?

Are his morale and health good, adequate or poor?

THE EFFECTS OF "CRAMMING" FOR THE TESTS

It has happened rarely—only twice or thrice over several years—that one has felt a candidate has been primed about a task. On such occasions, rather than help it seemed to handicap: to show him to poor advantage by inhibiting his spontaneity. It is of course possible that those one suspected were the unsuccessful dissimulators.

A point to note is that candidates are never told what are the correct or optimum solutions of any task: they are told that there are a variety of ways in which the task can be satisfactorily completed: which is of course true. An even more important point is that knowing a functional solution, it still has to be carried out: the need for group-cohesiveness still remains and this may even be complicated by pre-knowledge. A third point is that there should always be a variety of alternative tasks (if only to maintain an experimental creative frame of mind in the observer team). A fourth and important point is that a task is only one item in a variegated and balanced pattern of testing.

This problem hardly seems to arise in practice: though it is occasionally mentioned by those with little knowledge or appreciation of the theory and spirit of this type of procedure. Even specific cramming on the general principles of group-effectiveness —while they should impart an intellectual appreciation of good social behaviour which might eventually fertilise the spirit and bloom into action—could not help the deliberate dissimulator under the calculated and distributed stresses of the Stress Group Task. After all, the whole object is to elicit social behaviour which is spontaneous and natural: in so far as it fails to do just that, it has failed in its purpose.

EVALUATING GROUP-EFFECTIVENESS

THE GABI RANK-RATING

The practical purpose of the Leaderless Group or Stress Group task is to evaluate the level of each candidate's group effectiveness (GE). This may be expressed in terms of relative or absolute level i.e. by ranking or rating the group.

To rank a group is to arrange its members in the order of their GE. Thus:—

$$2\ 8\ 7\ 3\ 1\ 5\ 4\ 6$$

indicates that 2 put up the best performance, 8 the next best and 6 the worst. Ranking does not however indicate their absolute level: even the best candidate may have made a poor contribution, or even the worst a good one.

To rate a candidate is to express his GE in terms of an absolute or fixed standard i.e. good, adequate, borderline or inadequate. To rate a group is to arrange them in terms of these standards.

After a time, one devised a simple and practical means of simultaneously ranking and rating a group which simplified one's work considerably and largely replaced the recording devices described in Chapter IX (though these are indispensable in one's apprenticeship observing). It is based on a 4-point rating of Good, Adequate, Borderline and Inadequate: for mnemonic purposes one may term it the "GABI" rank-rating.

After ranking the candidates as above, one divides them into 4 sub-groups by inserting 2 dots and a stroke (. . /) between the figures. One way of doing it is to arrange and rearrange the candidates' numbers on 4 lines or levels until one reaches a satisfying final formulation: this may then be expressed on a single line by means of the 2 dots and a stroke.

The following rank-rating

$$.\ .\ 2\ 8\ 7\ 3\ /\ 1\ 5\ 4\ 6$$

indicates that 2, 8, 7 and 3 were borderline in that order and the rest inadequate. No performance was adequate and the best merely borderline.

This rank-rating

$$.\ 2\ 8\ 7\ .\ 3\ 1\ /\ 5\ 4\ 6$$

indicates that 2, 8 and 7 were adequate, 3 and 1 borderline and

the rest inadequate. The group is therefore quite a good one.
A rank-rating

$$2\ 8\ .\ 7\ 3\ .\ 1\ 5\ /\ 4\ 6$$

would indicate an excellent or brilliant group.

If there is reason to doubt a man's stability—whatever his
rating—this may be indicated by a question-mark above his
number or by underlining or circling it. Or one may, more
elaborately, indicate queries about level, group-cohesiveness or
stability by three different modes of marking the number.

This simple formula, easily expressed, and requiring not even
pencil or paper, simultaneously indicates:

1 the *ranking* or relative level of each candidate
2 the *rating* or absolute level of each candidate
3 the quality or *collective level* of the group in whose context
  he has been tested.
4 the *Query candidates* i.e. those who are borderline or question-
  marked for stability, etc.

A simple rank-rating of this kind makes for precision in
observation, judgement and recording. It prevents judgement
deteriorating, as it too easily may, into a vague impressionistic
guessing of each man's level as either "OK" or "useless", and
can be applied to any small group anywhere.

ITS POSSIBLE USES

It lends itself to the following important uses.

1 It enables one *to compare a candidate* (a) *in different tests* or
fields of activity (b) *at different phases* in the testing procedure;
one's own routine practice was to take 3 rank-ratings (i) Group
Discussion (GD), (ii) Progressive Group Task (PGT) and (iii)
Final Exercise (FE).

With regard to (a), it is useful to compare a man's effectiveness in discussion (i) with that on a practical job (ii). The homo-
geneity or heterogeneity of level in different fields will throw
some light on the degree to which a personality is balanced in
a stable manner. Gross discrepancy will suggest a query for
investigation.

With regard to (b), it is useful to compare effectiveness in
the BS (i and ii) with that in the FE (iii). It was usual for the
immature (NY), the inhibited and the slow-starters to improve
with time and to rank higher in the FE than in the BS: often

they emerged from their shells only at the very end. The "thrusters" and "group-disruptives" tend to deteriorate with time.

2 It provides a communicable recordable formula which enables observers *to compare* or pool their *rank-ratings* at any "screening" i.e. Query Conference, Final Board etc. A comparison of rank-ratings may suggest queries about candidates of whom there are discrepant opinions. By pooling individual rank-ratings to form an agreed team GABI rank-rating, the team is compelled to pool its collective knowledge. One found it invaluable as a means of pooling the collective observations of the psychological department.

It facilitates the development and maintenance of common Board standards and norms, without which a Board cannot hope to arrive at cooperative judgements of consistent quality.

It will also assist in the indoctrination and training and testing of new team members in these norms and standards. It is a constant check on—as well as guide to—the judgements of team members without in any way inhibiting these judgements. As there will always of necessity be weaker and stronger members, more experienced and less, it will provide a clue to the personal equation of each and an index to the amount of "weighting" by the President that his opinions will need at the Final Board etc.

3 A third possible use is *to compare one's own final rank-rating (or that of the team) with the group's choice as "Leader"* in the "Test of Objective Judgement" *and with the rankings of individual candidates.* This provides a relative assessment of the collective judgement of the group, and of the judgement of each individual member, that one found of particular value and interest. Chapter xvii points out some of the interesting implications, possibilities and lines for investigation.

4 A fourth use—implicit in the formula—is *to dissociate the collective level of the group from the individual levels of its members.* Already in this chapter one has mentioned a possible source of fallacy in a carry-over of "halo" or "horn" from the group to its members.

GROUP REPORTAGE: A SAMPLE

A useful reportage of the entire group will be provided by a GABI rank-rating plus a list of queries about each member: a *proforma* for a pooled team version of this is suggested in Chapter XI as a useful way of focussing the Query Conference.

Below is a sample of this type of reportage: in this case it is a combined report on the complete BS i.e. discussion and task:—

8 . . 2 3 7 / 1 6 4 5

This group is very unequal: there is one very good candidate, the others are borderline or inadequate.

8 outstanding: not over-dominant, no obvious queries.

2 much drive, energy and keenness: some weakness in planning, possibly due to limited intelligence and education. Level?

3 good intelligence and education but lacks drive: is anxious and tries too hard: seems slightly "shut-in" with poorish social contact. Contact? Shut-in? Stability?

7 his intelligence, education and background are good enough but he is not showing very much: seems immature and shy. Immaturity? He may come out. (Watch in Command Situations).

1 shows only slight low-level participation. Level?

6 of extremely high intelligence and superior education but at the moment seems extremely inhibited and "shut-in", driveless and rather "wet". Shut-in??? Stability???

4 very immature: might possibly improve in the later phases or show up better in the interview. Immaturity???

5 much drive and energy but tactless and egocentric; apparently compensating for a limited intelligence: tends to disrupt the group's effort. Group-disruptive? Stability?

Providing as it does a provisional estimate of each man's group-effectiveness and queries about factors that may subtract from it, it will be seen that a reportage of this kind can be a useful contribution to the Query Conference: and that a team version of it will set very precisely the queries that Phase 2 is required to answer.

CHAPTER XI

THE QUERY CONFERENCE OR FIRST INTERPHASE SCREEN

Perhaps the most profitable 5–10 minutes in the entire board procedure is the Query Conference (QC) held informally after the BS. Into it is distilled the quintessential drop of pooled wisdom that has accrued to the observer team from:—

a a screening of the "background" and "projective" material,
b the CO's report with its estimate of the candidate's level and its queries if any,
c the BS.

Into the QC converge these 3 streams; a critical screening and analysis of factual and written material, a report on the candidate's recent adjustment to the Army, and observation in the field by 3 or more observers. There they are co-ordinated into a provisional team estimate of each candidate's group-effectiveness (GE) and a team list of queries about factors that may subtract from that GE. The team estimate is taken by each observer to Phase 2 as a hypothesis to be tested and either confirmed, modified or rebutted; the team queries are referred to the specific tests or interviews in that phase most likely to resolve them.

A point worth keeping in mind is that while queries should be formulated as clearly and definitely as possible, estimates of level should be left as fluid as possible until the Board makes its last and final decision.

TO GET THE RIGHT ANSWER, ONE MUST PUT THE RIGHT QUESTION

As the field of personality is large and procedure time limited, it is important to get down, as early as possible, to the critical query areas in each candidate's personality. A judgement is the answer to a question and to get a clear answer you must put a clear question. The purpose of the QC is to put the right questions so that the remainder of the procedure may be made to yield the right answers.

How then raise the right questions?

By pooling all the data, impressions, opinions and queries up-to-date: by noting similarities and dissimilarities, agreements and discrepancies: by regarding every discrepancy of opinion, every shared doubt as a query for the next testing phase. It is the holding of every discrepancy and doubt in the filter through which the pooled material passes that constitutes the QC as an interphase screen, sieve or filter. Its result is to so concentrate and narrow the field of enquiry in Phase 2 that the observer team may focus all its resources intensively on the query areas in each candidate's personality.

DISCUSS THE GROUP FIRST, THEN ITS MEMBERS

It is best to consider the group first: its general collective level, whether good, adequate, borderline or inadequate; then the chronological events and phases of the task: the impasses and how met by group and individual: whether it functioned cohesively as a unit, was clique-directed or dominated by an individual, or was inchoate and never achieved any organisation.

Its members may then be considered individually: from the best downwards (using a team GABI rank-rating). Experience suggests it is best to discuss, first the candidate's GE in the BS, then the CO's report, followed by queries raised in the paper screening. At this stage the Sjt-testers should, one feels, be brought "into the picture": one's reasons are given in Chapter XIX.

A TEAM PROFORMA FOR RANK-RATINGS AND QUERIES

A useful technical device for helping the QC to use its information, experience and skill to maximum effect would be a small proforma or slip for each observer as described below. This is a modification, for team purposes, of a technique one found invaluable.

The upper half would contain the observer's GABI rank-rating of the BS: below it, the agreed team rank-rating. This might be preceded by two lines: one to note the CO's report and queries, another possibly to note Pointer queries.

The lower half would have 8 lines, one for each candidate in the order of his rank-rating. Across the page from left to right, each line might be sub-divided into 3 columns (besides that for the candidate's number): the first for queries about level, the second about group-cohesiveness, the third about stability. Those for referral to the medical psychologist might be starred.

Such a proforma compels a clear and precise formulation of one's estimate of the BS and one's queries up to date and leaves little scope for impressionism.

THE QC SHOULD BE INFORMAL AND SPONTANEOUS

As an informal conference—most of whose value is due to its encouraging complete spontaneity of utterance in each observer, whatever his rank, age or capacity—it should not be conducted or directed by a chairman: though the team leader may watch to see that a routine minimal procedure is followed and its essential spirit maintained. It should however be a "sit-down" conference: a conference so informal that it is conducted on the field inevitably degenerates into no conference at all.

The President—because of his function as impartial judge at the Final Board—should take no part: though he may be present to inform himself of the efficient running of the board. But whether his role be judicial or participant, it is important that such influence as accrues from his seniority, rank and force of personality should serve to loosen the team into spontaneity and not to dominate it into rigidity, inflexibility and ossification of the mind.

Any attempt to force the order of discussion—especially in terms of rank—is against the spirit of collective team judgement and likely to weaken or paralyse the contributions of junior or less articulate members.

It is important at this stage to resist the temptation to argue about queries or attempt to resolve them instead of merely mentioning them, along with the behaviour which has suggested them. One should take special note of queries not raised by oneself or not corresponding to one's own first impressions.

QUERIES ABOUT LEVEL

Intelligence and education have already indicated the candidate's potential functional level. Further queries are referred mainly to the Command Situations, the Planning Project and the interviews.

The candidate's self-identification with the field for which he is being selected will be investigated in the interviews. A good Interests Session should throw considerable light on it. The Apparatus Session (page 118) is prototypic of a type of test devised to project more precisely this identification with the job:

further developments in this direction should be of increasing value in professional, technical and administrative fields.

QUERIES ABOUT GROUP-COHESIVENESS

Group-cohesiveness is observed in every group situation, leaderless or otherwise: but specific queries are referred to the Human Problems Session and, where they are at all serious, to the psychiatric interview for an exploration in depth into their psychodynamics.

But the Human Problems Session, conducted as in Chapter XIII, will throw light on most queries of this kind. One found, in practice, that they revolved round 4 or 5 man-management and group-management roles which are fully discussed in that chapter but will merely be listed here:—

1. *Empathy* i.e. the ability to have—and to convey—a sympathetic understanding of the emotional reactions and needs of others:
2. *Encouragement* i.e. the ability to raise morale and encourage group-cohesive attitudes in individuals and groups:
3. *Firmness* i.e. the ability to reprimand or take a strong line when it is indicated and to discourage group-disruptive attitudes:
4. *Tact* i.e. the ability to combine (3) with (2)—reprimand with "face-saving":
5. *"Bringing others into the Picture"* i.e. the ability to relate others emotionally to the common purpose and to make them feel they have a part to play in reference to it.

The first four of these roles are concerned with binding the members of a group to each other: the fifth is concerned with binding the whole group to a common purpose.

QUERIES ABOUT STABILITY

One's own experience is that 1 in 4 of any group of men and women are complex—so far as selection for a job is concerned—and need careful placement and handling. About one-half of these are not generally realised to be so.

Many of these would—and do—make excellent leaders under favourable circumstances. Many of the finest leaders are probably so because they elect to live, necessarily unstably, on their very highest functional level: well above their level of optimum stability and comfort. These successful ones are probably the emergent tip of the iceberg and the vast majority of such types need careful handling if they are to realise their potentialities and rise above water.

While it is not the function of the non-medical observer to diagnose instability, he should learn to recognise the "red light" which suggests referral for psychiatric check-up. Co-operating with an experienced medical psychologist on the same board, he can learn to do so. The Spectrum Rating embodies the commoner types of "complex" candidate that kept cropping up over the several years of its use. Most of the "complex 25 per cent" will fall *in some degree* into one or other of these six types:—

1 The candidate prone to "psychosomatic complaints" (see p. 59). He may have a long record of minor complaints with exacerbations at exams, new jobs, etc. Under stress he will make the most of minor symptoms of a physical nature i.e. fatigue, headache, dyspepsia, muscular pains, etc. His Spectrum Rating is Indigo B1.

2 The candidate showing marked anxiety with little or no apparent cause: or obsessional-compulsive (i.e. self-driving) traits. These types are closely related and shade into one other: the latter is probably the more intelligent, more conscientious, more ambitious type who attempts persistently to compensate for his anxiety and sense of inadequacy by continuous self-driving. He may drive others as he drives himself. His Spectrum Rating is Indigo B2.

3 The candidate of strong but antisocial drive, disruptive and difficult: though not psychopathic, he could become so under stress. His Spectrum Rating is Indigo A6.

The next three types are easily confused because all may seem shy: they are however quite different types with quite different potentialities.

4 The shy candidate, socially a "slow starter" because of sheer youth or lack of social experience. He is rated NY (Not Yet i.e. immature) and if his level and identification with the job are sufficiently high, he may do very well: especially if the training period can be lengthened or modified to assist his development.

5 The shyness of the socially inhibited "cycloid" type, whose emotionality is labile and prone to mood swings. His Spectrum Rating is Indigo B3.

6 The "shut-in" or schizoid aloof type of candidate: rated Indigo B4.

It is especially important to distinguish the last two.

The shy inhibited cycloid is intensely interested in people, extremely sensitive to the group and very empathic. He is pathetically keen to participate: extravagantly elated if he succeeds, profoundly depressed if he fails. Quite a large proportion of brilliant but somewhat unstable leaders are of this type. Careful direction and training may stabilise them and should at any rate ensure a useful contribution to the community: badly handled they become disruptive mischief-makers or depressed misfits.

The "shut-in" or schizoid personality is another story. He does not particularly seek or need company and may genuinely prefer to be "alohn"; he is socially apathetic, indifferent or detached rather than inhibited or shy. In so far as he is disinterested in people, it is not easy for him to acquire great skill in man-management or group-management roles. He may however—if his level is sufficiently high—do well or brilliantly in a specially chosen technical or professional field where the need for social contact is reduced to a minimum.

The term "shut-in" (which aptly describes the detachment of the schizoid personality—as if separated from the warmth of humanity by a pellicle of cellophane) should not be used for the previous two types i.e. the shyness of the immature or the inhibited seclusiveness of the discouraged. If the medical psychologist is to help a selection board to become more sensitively aware of the gamut and range of human personality, he must discourage the imprecise use of words so expressively helpful as this.

REFERRALS TO THE PSYCHOLOGICAL DEPARTMENT FOR INTERVIEW

After much experience of screening groups psychologically, the impression left is that while in an ideal selection procedure, every candidate should be psychologically "vetted" in an interview, in practice 50 per cent *might* usefully and 25 per cent *should* clearly be interviewed by a medical psychologist. That is to say, while all should undergo a paper screening, two candidates in every group of 8 are sufficiently complex to warrant an expert medico-psychological opinion on their placement and disposal. Moreover *only such a screening, interpreted by a medical psychologist* with subsequent opportunities for observation, *will indicate clearly which 25 per cent* of the group *should be interviewed.*

In a board of the WOSB type, the best working procedure would be a system of graded priorities. The medical psychologist would interview 25 per cent: to include not only the difficult personality problems but also a percentage of the most outstanding candidates. For reasons fully discussed in Chapter XIV, one's own practice was to interview the best candidate in each batch and every candidate of outstanding quality or unusually high potential level: these constituted about 10 per cent of one's interviews. The next priority of 25 per cent—to include candidates with moderate personality problems or of borderline level so far as intelligence and education are concerned—would be interviewed by the general psychologist. The remaining 50 per cent would have a 5-minute "educational and vocational" check-up—to check, complete and amplify where necessary, their questionnaires by the Sjt-testers or equivalent junior psychologists.

All these interviews should be closely linked and under the supervision of the medical psychologist, who has had by far the widest clinical experience of men under stress. Candidates who proved more complex or difficult than at first apparent would be referred up the scale of experience for further discussion or re-interview.

A full-length psychological interview of each candidate by one man in a 3-day procedure would be an impossible burden. A short interview of each would in one's opinion be of limited value. The system of priorities would make possible:—

a A thorough and complete screening of the entire batch.
b A more intensive investigation of the major personality problems for the guidance and further instruction of the board.
c The fullest use, training and participation of the whole psychological team. General psychologists must have clinical experience of men—and a means of relating observed behaviour with emotional attitudes and motivation as revealed in interview—if their contributions to a selection board are to be of value.

d The lightening of the medical psychologist's load in this way will add immeasurably to his efficiency.

Occasionally it has been objected that selective interviewing by the medical psychologist will make the candidate feel he is being discriminated against, and that this is bad. If he so feels, it is bad. In one's own experience, this only occurred—or may have occurred—on the occasions when one was unable to take the very simple necessary measures. The group-talk given on Day 1 pointed out in some detail the possible reasons for interview. Moreover complex candidates are not rarer on the higher levels of ability: they may even be commoner. One's practice of interviewing outstanding candidates made this clear. Also, in the group talk, one offered to interview any candidate who might not be selected for psychological interview but desired one.

If these simple explanations are reinforced by the President in his introductory talk and by other observers in their informal contacts with candidates: if negative suggestion is avoided in explanations: if in addition the medical psychologist does make a point of being helpful in some way to those he interviews (as suggested in Chapter xiv), no feeling of discrimination need arise. Candidates are not slow to appreciate an attitude of frankness and integrity: and are not unappreciative of any help one may be able to give. One's own comparatively large sampling of the younger generation indicates that their prejudices are not necessarily those of their elders.

PHASE 2: THE OBSERVER TEAM SPLITS

CHAPTER XII

DIFFERENTIATING GROUP-EFFECTIVENESS INTO ITS COMPONENT ROLES: THE PSO BATTERY AND INTERVIEWS

The Query Conference has pooled the results of Phase 1 to form:—

a a team provisional estimate of each candidate's GE (Group-effectiveness),

b a team list of queries about factors that may subtract from that GE.

The object of Phase 2 is:—

a to differentiate his GE into its component roles so that they may be examined more closely and the queries resolved. Queries about level are referred especially to the Planning Project, Command Situations, interviews etc. Queries about group-cohesiveness are referred to the Human Problems Session and are considered in all leaderless group tests, the interview, etc. Queries about stability are referred to the medical psychologist. Queries about motivation and identification with the military field are considered especially in the Human Problems Session and the interviews.

b to split the observer team and differentiate it into its members functioning as specialists. The PSO conducts the "PSO Battery": the team leader, medical psychologist (and occasionally a technical PSO) conduct their interviews.

A FURTHER NOTE ON GROUP-COHESIVENESS

Leadership is a collective function: collective in the sense that it is the integrated synergised expression of a group's efforts: it can only arise in relation to a group problem or purpose: it is not the sum of individual dominances and contributions, it is their relationship. ·

In so far as a man contributes to the collective leadership function, he does so by relating every member of the group functionally and emotionally with the group purpose. It is especially important that he relate them emotionally and that he increase their self-identification with it. In so doing, he will ask the group to serve—not the personal dominance of a single leader—but the common purpose, the challenge to the group, the "Law of the Total Situation" (LOTS): and will demand loyalty—not to himself—but to that purpose.

He will realise that the ultimate authority and true sanction for leadership, at every point where it is exercised, resides—not in the individual, however dominant or strong or efficient he may be—but in the "total situation" and in the demands of that situation i.e. the Law of the Total Situation. It is the situation that creates the imperative, not the individual. To the extent that the individual is aware of that imperative, is able to make others aware of it, is able to make them willing to serve it: to the extent that he is able to release collective capacities and emotional attitudes that may be related fruitfully to the solution of the group's problems: to that extent he is exercising leadership.

He will realise that a two-fold link—functional *and* emotional —between the group and the LOTS is implicit in any leadership that is effective: and that it is this two-fold link that makes leadership inevitably a collective function in which human drives and human abilities and skills are harnessed to cooperate with the environment.

THE PSO BATTERY

THE COMMAND SITUATION (CS)

Because candidates were being selected for a military field, the situations consisted of practical projects of graduated difficulty, putting stress on different roles in group-effectiveness i.e. on planning the solution of a difficult problem, on organising the group in a task of some detail, on controlling its members in a finicky job, on working patiently on a slow job or with precision at a fast tempo, etc.

The tasks were like the individual obstacles in the PGT i.e. moving heavy, unwieldy or delicate burdens—or the group itself—over walls, streams, trees, etc. But the theory of the test (to differentiate GE into some of its component roles) does not of course necessitate practical projects: provided there is a group to handle and a problem to solve, it does not matter what the nature of the task. For non-military fields (administrative, executive, managerial) other situations can and should be devised: possibly similar to the Human Problems discussed in the next chapter; but with a group to deal with and not merely one man i.e. the stooge.

Technique

For a group of 8, the choice of a dozen situations (5–20 minutes, averaging 15) is sufficient. One CS is pre-selected for each candidate and before it is due, he is detached from the group, shown the task and given a few minutes to prepare his plan. Ordinarily he is briefed to stand apart from the group—who are not to prompt him or contribute to the plan—and to direct them without taking any practical part, except perhaps to explain or demonstrate. This will discourage the brighter candidates from doing his CS for him.

In one variant of the technique (based apparently on a misconception), the briefing gave no indication whether he might participate: and it was considered a good sign if he showed willingness to "muck-in".

There are two strong objections:—

1 One should already have learnt from the BS sufficient of his willingness to participate (a main function of the BS is to elicit just this).

2 It is not necessarily good leadership to "muck in": the BS will have indicated whether he is ready to do so where this is helpful. The situations are so designed not to need for their solution the push-pulling powers of one additional man, but to elicit capacity for planning the problem and handling the group. Moreover one of the commonest faults, if not *the* commonest, of the borderline or low-level candidate is that he will "muck-in" and try to do the job himself because he cannot either plan the solution or organise the group. "Mucking in" is one of the commonest ways of concealing incompetence and inability either to give proper instructions or see them carried out.

Pre-selecting the CS for the Query Candidate

The easiest tasks may be given to those who will clearly not make the grade, so as not to discourage them or disturb the balance of the group. Those who will clearly make the grade may be given easy tasks but it may be advisable to give an outstanding candidate a difficult one so as not to discourage the others.

The candidate of borderline level may be set a problem of some complexity: the timid submissive one may be set a task which demands sufficient firmness to give crisp, clear and quick directions. The impetuous somewhat irresponsible candidate may be required to exercise care, precision, deliberation and persistence in the face of frustration: the lethargic candidate, whose "drive" is queried, may be given a task requiring dash and expedition.

Occasionally one may set a task which is practically impossible or extremely difficult although not realised to be so: where one particularly wishes to be definite about a candidate's reaction to frustration i.e. in the suspect bully who may drive and blame others when under stress.

Comparing Performance in the BS and CS

A man may have the urge to leadership and responsibility but not the capacity: or the capacity but not the urge. The CS aims to elicit leadership capacity which may not have been manifest in the BS.

When there are very strong candidates in a group, a man of lesser but sufficient ability may not reveal it because opportunity has not presented itself. There are others who can function on a sufficiently high level if compelled to do so; but who lack the mature sense of responsibility or the confidence—through sheer immaturity, inexperience or even genuine modesty—to seek responsibility and leadership on their own appropriate level.

There are responsibility-seekers and responsibility-accepters: the latter will accept it but will not seek it. By giving the candidate a problem to solve and a group to handle, one hopes to reveal the inhibited, shy, modest or lazy responsibility-accepters as well as the lesser leaders who may be responsibility-seekers but whose ability has been cloaked by that of stronger men.

A point which may be mentioned is the opportunity provided by the CS to observe a man's followership and loyalty, his willingness and ability to cooperate with—and follow—the vested leadership of another. On some able but disruptive types, this may constitute a sore demand, a considerable stress and a high test.

SELECTIVE OBSTACLES (SO)

Technique

In theory, this was a test of a man's ability to plan the use of his body and his muscular skills: *not* a test of athleticism, stamina or physical courage. Those who hoped it would give a pointer to the existence of "guts" found it disappointing. Tasks which demanded a tolerance for heights were particularly misleading as an index to courage and were ultimately discarded.

An obstacle course of 10–12 graduated athletic tasks was laid out over a limited area: it included leaps, rope-climbing, cat-walking on elevated planks, long jumps, balancing, etc., and each was given a score from 1 to 10 marked on a board beside it. The object was to score as many points as one could in three minutes. The candidates did not witness each other's performance and the competitive element did not enter.

The group was given 3–5 minutes to make a preliminary silent "recce" of the course so that each could decide on his plan of action: they were then taken out of sight of the task, recalled one by one and given three minutes to carry out the plan.

Each might be quizzed before his attempt: on the obstacles he proposed to take, his order of taking them and the score he hoped to make. Afterwards he might be quizzed about changes he may have made in his plan and why: and whether, if required to repeat the task, he would alter his plan in any way, etc.

An occasional modification was to give the candidate a message of brain-twisting tortuosity to memorise, which he was expected to repeat after his attempt. As a device to assist a splitting of the personality this might have been excellent: but there seemed to be no medico-psychological justification for regarding it as a test of character, persistence or stability.

Interpretation

This was the most dramatic but probably the least valuable test in the procedure. One of the first that boards, especially the purely military members on them, felt inclined to disregard or drop, or to regard as an interim relaxation for candidates and observers.

One must admit to a fondness for the test despite its great limitations. While it made no consistently regular contribution, it did seem to provide occasional useful pointers. One felt that it might have been more valuable if

a the "halo" or "horn" of physical fitness and athletic skill could have been discounted.

b it were more closely related to the rest of the testing procedure

c more attention were paid to certain points.

In one's own experience, the following three points are worthy of note:—

1 The amount of planning and judgement shown in distributing effort among the limbs, in balancing rope-climbing with jumping, muscular effort with feats of coordination etc.: also in relating one's plan to one's physical equipment and skill: the non-athletic would aim, unless he lacked judgement, at a lesser performance than the star athlete.

2 The man's level of aspiration as indicated by comparing his plan with his actual achievement. Some were too sanguine in wild over-compensation for a fancied inferiority: others were reckless to a fault or over-cautious to the point of "fragility": others made a self-estimate which was reasonably objective in relation to skill and experience. It was also valuable to note the man's capacity for objectively judging his own performance.

3 Pointers to the accident-prone, the "unlucky", the awkward, the over-compensators of borderline intelligence who might become "doom-merchants": and any who might become a danger to themselves and others if required to operate in a physical *milieu* or above a limited level. One felt that the SO test ¦did often suggest these at a glance. Sometimes by such pointers as: conspicuous absence of easy natural body movement and balance, awkwardness linked with anxious tension, the occasional individual with an unusual and crippling lack of physical courage, etc.

Value

The importance of physical qualities in excess of ordinary physical fitness for a job may easily be overemphasised, and there seems to be no evidence that morale or leadership quality continue to grow with any such increment.

Even in the military field and in the "teeth" arms, it is doubtful if a Selection Board can learn more about the influence on leadership level of the physical factors than can be obtained from:—

a the very complete PULHEEMS system of medical categorising to ensure a man reaches the required physical standard:
b a medical screening by the Board's medical psychologist.

In non-military fields, an appropriate and comprehensive medical investigation of physical fitness should cover all the physical factors that may influence leadership function, morale and stability.

THE INTERESTS SESSION (IS)

It was found convenient to hold this while candidates were waiting turn to be interviewed by the interviewing members. Before the session, they were shown the rooms where they would be interviewed and told the order: each left the session quietly when due for interview and returned equally quietly when it was over.

Technique

The group should sit, as in the UGD, in a square or circle round a low coffee-table covered with large ashtrays.

The simplest technique is to ask each member to give a 5-minute Job Talk, Hobby Talk, or a talk on any subject he chooses to the rest of the group. They are given 5 minutes to prepare (the shortness of the notice diminishes apprehensive anticipation and helps spontaneity) and are to speak seated and in any order. The order of speaking, whether early or late, may provide pointers.

An improvement is to brief the group to get into a huddle and arrange among themselves what each will discuss with a view to providing a session of interesting talks. After or during each talk, the group may question, heckle or criticise the speaker. This technique provides (a) a preliminary huddle phase (b) the talks (c) group response to the talks.

A still further technical advance is to allow the PSO, if sufficiently competent and experienced, to interrupt or intervene in either of the previous procedures and to ask anybody anything at any time. This constitutes a group interview by the PSO (see p. 129). As in all interviewing, he must project the personalities of those interviewed while effacing his own: and must relax, stimulate or provoke them into spontaneity (unlike the UGD, one is concerned not so much with their effectiveness in discussion as with its content and with the nature of their interests). He may bring out the inhibited candidate by asking "Well, No. 5, what is your feeling about this?": or stimulate the group generally by enquiring "Does anyone know the answer to this—has anyone a suggestion?" etc.

Linking it with the Human Problems Session (HPS)

What strikes one as an optimum procedure would be the IS immediately followed by the HPS. The former would warm up and loosen the proceedings and lead to a very spontaneous easy projection of interpersonal attitudes in the latter. Moreover the individual appearing before the group in the IS would lead easily into the Officer and Stooge (as a pair) of the HPS revealing their attitudes to the group.

And with the UGD

It is intensely interesting to note the progressive revelation of personality from the UGD through the IS to the HPS. The first gives a line on spontaneity and group-cohesiveness and may reveal something about the range and nature of interests: the IS will amplify the interests, the HPS will round off the picture of the candidate's essential group-cohesiveness. This progression is equivalent to the progression—in the practical type of task— from the leaderless group of the PGT to the Command Situations. Together with the interview, these 3 tests should answer most queries about the candidate's interests and social attitudes.

THE HUMAN PROBLEMS SESSION (HPS)

This will be discussed in the next chapter.

THE PLANNING PROJECT (PP)

This is a "work-sample" test which projects individual planning and organising ability as well as group-cohesiveness in a committee setting. Its value is easily recognised and it is likely to undergo considerable further development as a test for potential administrative or managerial ability.

The technique here described is an intriguing combination of an individual with a group project: in two parts of ¾–1 hour, separated if possible by a "break" for tea. Shortened versions (20–30 minutes) and extended versions (several days) for special purposes have been experimented with.

The group is given a project and each member is given a dossier containing details, maps, inventory of materials available and a general outline of the conditions under which it is to be carried out. They are required to consider the project individually and devise their plans; then meet in committee to arrive at a common plan of action.

Types of project used were: reorganising quickly a town recently disorganised by battle and now behind the battle line: planning a pleasure camp or island, a youth camp, a large school, a training unit for delinquent young soldiers, etc., etc. In some projects, members of the group might be given special functions i.e. Town Major, RE Officer, medical officer, etc. This is useful where the PSO wishes to test candidates specifically in certain roles. But on the whole, the better plan is to leave to the group the initiative in allocating functions. A chairman should never be chosen for the group: nor should it be suggested that they elect one.

Phase 1 is an individual project: each member studies his dossier and prepares his written plan: this is taken from him after Phase 2 and will indicate (a) the quality of his planning (b) the use he has made of it in Phase 2.

Phase 2 is a leaderless group situation: the candidates sit round a table with their written plans and proceed to work out their common plan in committee. One can observe about each his ability to view objectively the pooled ideas, to coordinate them and to get his ideas "over" in committee i.e. his planning and organising abilities and his group-cohesiveness.

One man will make excellent plans but fail to convince the group: another will carry them with an inferior plan: still another will seize on the plans of others and attempt to get credit for them. The better leader will evaluate objectively both his own ideas and those of others: he will select and coordinate the best of them and give credit to each for his contribution. By comparing his written plans with his performance in Phase 2 one will note how well he planned and what use he was able to make of it.

In Chapter v, level of functioning was considered in terms of

3 phases i.e. planning, organising and practical execution. One could make of the Planning Project a 3-phase project, in which the third phase would be the actual practical task. One would then have a first phase of individual planning, a second phase of group planning and organising and a third phase of collective action. It would of necessity have to be a simpler project.

A PGT was tried with some success at 10 WOSB in 1944 in which a preliminary phase of committee planning was followed by the actual practical task i.e. the second and third phase of the 3-phase task suggested above (a first phase of individual planning was omitted). That is to say, the group was given the written details of a practical task along with the materials available for use and were directed to discuss their plan in committee before carrying it out.

THE APPARATUS SESSION (AS)

Significance

Among the many experiments in testing procedure made by WOSB, of especial interest were some preliminary essays in projecting "engineering personality" in an "Apparatus Session". This was incorporated in Boards whose special purpose was to select schoolboys for Engineering Cadetships to be held for 12–18 months at a University. After which, either they were to be diverted to one of the Services for commission in a technical branch (in the Army after passing another WOSB) or directed to civilian engineering posts.

The importance of the "Apparatus Session" is that it does suggest a basis for the projective testing of special interests and attitudes in different professional fields. It may well be proto-typic of the test that will help to select junior leaders in special fields, and those likely to benefit from special types of professional training.

Rationale

The rationale of the AS was to get an assessment of a man's interest and feeling for technical apparatus by observing his behaviour in a setting of such equipment: how he manipulated mechanical, electrical and optical apparatus: the questions he put to the technical expert in attendance: the sort of information he was able to elicit: his attitudes as revealed by an informal chat in that setting.

The aim was definitely not to ascertain his mechanical

aptitude, his comparative "ham-handedness" with apparatus or his knowledge of physics, mechanics, etc. It was to project his interest in these things and whether it was sufficient—provided his general level of intelligence and education were adequate—to enable him after training to function on leadership or professional level.

Technique

The AS lasted about 40 minutes and was conducted by the PSO and Psychological Officer or Sgt-Tester. Initially a highly trained technical officer was enlisted to give both of them sufficient knowledge of the apparatus to enable them—with the help of technical briefing notes—to rate performance. It was considered they could do this without a profound technical knowledge. It does however seem advisable that the PSO for this purpose should come from a technical arm. At least one of the observers should have a specialised knowledge of the field for which they are selecting.

Pieces of mechanical, electrical, and optical apparatus were laid out on tables: such items as carburettor, magneto, sparking plug, binoculars, telescopes, etc. Four was the optimum number of candidates for each session and they were observed in the following 3 phases.

1 After a 5-minute briefing, 20 minutes were spent in allowing candidates to inspect, choose, examine and strip items that interested them. They were encouraged to ask as many questions as they wished and to these only direct answers were given. In an informal chat, the observers might enquire incidentally about a man's technical interests and hobbies. His general behaviour was noted: whether he felt at home and confident with apparatus or confused and fumbling: whether he found conversation a relief and escape from the apparatus: whether such a setting helped him in the informal interview or made him uncomfortable.

2 He was then asked to give a 5-minute talk to the group on the construction and operation of the item he chose: the description begun by one candidate might be finished by another who had handled a duplicate of the same item.

3 The last 10 minutes were devoted to a written questionnaire containing many brief questions of the multiple choice

E

type to which he ticked off appropriate answers. They were calculated to indicate his interest, reading and active participation in matters to do with cars, motor-cycles, boats, models, planes, etc. It included a short questionnaire in which, given a list of mechanical and other gadgets and a corresponding list of trade names and trade-marks, he was asked to link corresponding items.

Rating the AS

The two observers discussed their impressions and pooled their final estimate in a 4-point rating (i.e. $+2, +1, -1$, and -2) under the headings given below. They then agreed on a global rating, still in the 4-point scale, on the whole AS.

The headings were:—

1 *General Approach and Interest:* ranging from "keen and purposeful" to "casual and uninterested".
2 *Stripping and Assembly:* ranging from "shows confidence and competence", "selects different items" to "fumbling, confused, chooses the simplest items".
3 *Nature of Questions:* "purposeful" to "futile" or "no questions".
4 *Explanation:* "good grasp" to "no grasp".
5 *Predominant Trend of Interest:* whether mechanical, electrical, or optical and whether strongly or clearly indicated: any obvious lack of interest in certain fields was noted.

In selecting for leadership in a technical field, any estimate of the s factors—as distinct from the g factors in group-effectiveness—will usefully consider a test such as the AS along with the Interests Questionnaire and Interests Session (in so far as they throw light on special interests) and with the interview (in so far as it throws light on avowed ambitions and general motivation). Among the g factors, the OIR/ES level must come within the range of the level required by the job.

THE INTERVIEWS
GLOBAL ESTIMATES AND THEIR "WEIGHTING"

In later practice—from late 1945—the candidate was interviewed by the Team-leader and the medical psychologist (possibly assisted by the psychologist). The President's was a nominal

5-minute interview for purposes of check-up and recognition. In his judicial capacity, his opinion was required on the evidence and not on the candidate. In practice, this tended to become a useful additional opinion: the theoretical risk was that it might detract from the President's capacity to evaluate the evidence at the Final Board judicially, impartially and objectively. Practical reasons for preferring the participant President to the *deus ex machina* president are given on page 212. For certain Arms, a technical PSO interviewed the candidate to decide on his technical trainability for that Arm.

All the interviews except the last aimed at a global estimate of the candidate, though with a different "weighting" in each case. Allowance for this "weighting" would of course have to be made at the Final Board. The technical interview was never a global rating but considered technical trainability alone. The tendency was to replace it by "a technical vetting" by the Arm for which he was being considered: or by the remarkably efficient Attainments tests. These used a system of ticking off a choice of responses, could be carried out in a matter of minutes and seemed to correlate highly with the results of lengthier investigations. The most efficient procedure would seem to be the combination of

a "vetting" by the Arm,
b a check-up by Attainments tests carried out at WOSB,
c WOSB procedure modified for the special field.

So far as the interviewers' global estimates were concerned, the "weighting" in the medical psychologist's estimate would be on such factors as (a) degree of social maturation in relation to the expected norms for the candidate's age (b) the likely trend and tempo of immediate future maturation during the period of training and early commissioned service (c) the likely stability on the required level in that specific field.

The Team-leader "weighted" functional level and group-cohesiveness and their various sub-roles in their special bearing on the military field: also such factors as the compatibility of the candidate with a military background and setting, and his motivation or degree of identification with that field.

In so far as the President's interview went beyond the mere ability to recognise the candidate, he was likely to be interested in the last two points i.e. compatibility with a military field and emotional identification with it. The last two are of course not synonymous: a man may be identified but not compatible and *vice versa*.

THE DEVICE OF LINKED INTERVIEWS

It may be worth while mentioning here the useful auxiliary device of Linked Interviews. The results of testing may be linked not only through the interphase screens but also during the testing phase.

Specifically, there are occasions when one interviewer may wish to pass on newly discovered information or a new query to another interviewer who has not yet seen the candidate. It might be a query about stability to be referred to the medical psychologist: or a candidate suspected of being "bogus", dishonest or concealing something, where a fresh interviewer, once his attention is called to it, might elicit or confirm the truth by an approach from a different angle.

Occasionally an interviewer who has omitted to make an important enquiry may prefer to complete his data through the next interviewer rather than disconcert the candidate by recalling him.

THE ADVISABILITY IN PSYCHOLOGICAL MATTERS OF
TREADING SOFTLY

It is unfortunately too true that the non-psychological interviewer—once he has savoured the thrill of psychological enquiry —will rush in where even the most courageous and skilful medical psychologists would fear to tread. It is important that he should avoid intruding rudely into delicate personal and emotional topics where the medical psychologist would approach with the utmost professional circumspection and tact, or not at all, in a first interview.

As suggested on page 191, this may prevent the medical psychologist getting the data required for his own contribution to the Board: and he may have to spend his interview time striving to allay the emotional stir produced by his trespassing cooperator. It is right and inevitable that interviewers should with experience widen the scope of their enquiries; and it is desirable that they should increasingly appreciate the role of the emotions in social behaviour: but it is simple wisdom to tread carefully on the fringe of one's field.

CHAPTER XIII

THE HUMAN PROBLEMS SESSION

GENERAL COMMENTS

IT IS A PROJECTIVE SESSION

The Human Problems Session is a series of 8 stress interviews in which candidates—one as Officer, the other as Stooge or "other rank"—dramatise the handling of personal or disciplinary problems. Each candidate functions once as Officer and once as Stooge. The group sit round in a semi-circle and criticise and discuss the handling of each situation before going on to the next.

The ordinary problems that arise in any relationship between officer and subordinate, manager and employee are dramatised: and the purpose of the session is to induce each candidate to project his spontaneous social attitudes so that one may note his appreciation of interpersonal relationships, the degree of spontaneity and effective improvisation he is likely to show in handling them and the extent to which his own attitudes are naturally group-cohesive, group-disruptive, group-dependent or isolate.

As a result of queries—raised at the Query Conference or from the Personality Pointers—about his group-cohesiveness, general capacity for interpersonal relationships and aptitude in specific social roles, a specific Officer problem is pre-selected that may elicit the answer to these. A specific candidate is chosen to enact the Stooge role: and it is hoped that the subsequent stress interview will throw some light on the personalities of Officer and Stooge, but especially on the former.

WITH A STRESS ELEMENT

The stress is created by:—

1 giving the Officer only 30 seconds to prepare his plan of campaign i.e. as long as it takes him to read the card handed to him:

2 giving him 4 minutes to handle the problem as best he can; after which the interview can be—and usually is—terminated:

3 arranging the situation so that a clash of wills is inevitable and giving each only part of the facts:

4 pre-selecting both the Officer problem and the Stooge role to elicit the answer to a specific query.

THE GROUP ACTS AS A "SOCIAL RESONATOR"

In its original form, Officer interviewed Stooge before several observers without the presence of the group.   There was no discussion, no linkage of interviews, the emphasis rested very much on how the Officer handled his interview, and his spontaneity was not assisted by the high ratio of observers to observed. Under these conditions it was difficult for him to feel at ease or project his personality naturally.

The first group version that one knows of, was conducted by Major C. W. Robbins, SPSO, at 7 WOSB, Winchester in 1943. Interviews were conducted at a small table focussed in the centre of a semi-circle of candidates and each interview was criticised and discussed before passing on to the next.   By uniting the interviews in a series before the group and by briefing the candidates as described below, the individual interview ceased even to seem to be a measurable test—which it could never hope to be— but became a progressive projection *into* the group of the social attitudes of every member.

The presence of the group influences the session in at least three ways:—

1 It acts as a social resonator which intensifies the interaction between Officer and Stooge.

2 It produces a progressive rise in the emotional and social temperature of the group, a decrease in its social viscosity, an increasing animation and spontaneity and an increasingly fluid projection of each candidate's attitudes in:—

a his handling of the Officer problem
b his acting of the Stooge role
c his participation in the discussion
d his elicited responses to questions put by the PSO.

3 It permits of a Group Interview by the PSO who can discreetly interject questions addressed either to the group generally or to individual members.

The group inter-relationships are especially interesting: for we have the leaderless group background of the general discussion, the interaction of Officer and Stooge, the reaction of the Officer to his critics and the relationship between PSO and Group in the Group Interview aspect of the session.

A group technique of this kind when adequately conducted—and it does demand the minimal ability and training that the selectors of potential leaders must be expected to have—is a remarkable advance on the original version. The progressive spontaneity and happiness of the group must be seen to be believed, and persists after the session is over. Indeed the session is felt—as projective sessions should be—not as a test but as a pleasurable and illuminating experience which requires no "sealing off" despite the stresses it has created.

One's own conclusion—after being allowed to participate in many hundreds of these sessions at 7 WOSB Winchester, 10 WOSB Chester, and 5 WOSB Wormley—was that this was possibly the most valuable single technique in WOSB procedure. One which could give more useful information in a given time than any other: though, being but one item in the entire observational field, it must of course be related to the rest of the evidence. One which pointed the direction in which future technical development in the field of personality evaluation is likely to follow. *But, like every projective test, it cannot be conducted without psychological skill, or interpreted without psychological experience.*

The projective technique used here for selection and diagnostic purposes is similar to the "psychodramatic" technique devised by J. L. Moreno for therapeutic purposes. In these, individuals are encouraged to project their emotional attitudes by dramatising situations relevant to their own lives and problems: and by so doing, to gain an insight into their nature which may lead to their correction.

QUERIES ABOUT INTERPERSONAL RELATIONSHIPS ARE PINPOINTED

The session might be regarded as a "selective oral projection session" in that situations are pre-selected and the projection is in speech.

It is a technique for observing, under the microscope as it were, a man's group-cohesiveness, general capacity for interpersonal relationships and aptitude in specific social roles. If we continue the analogy, we may regard the Basic Series as the coarse adjustment of the microscope and the Human Problems Session as the fine adjustment: whose purpose is to pinpoint a specific area in the candidate's social personality to gain further, possibly even critical, information about that area.

This pinpointing is brought about not only by focussing on a pre-selected interpersonal problem but also by localising the relationship for the moment—in the interview part of the session —with only one other individual. The relationship becomes one of man-management rather than group-management.

THE TECHNIQUE OF CONDUCTING THE SESSION

TOPOGRAPHY AND LAY-OUT

Lay-out is important if one is to get a free cosy atmosphere in which the PSO can operate naturally and where observers may be felt, not as an intrusion, but as a mild social stimulant, an enhancement of the social resonator. An optimum arrangement is as follows: the 8 candidates are grouped in a horseshoe or semi-circle in the order of their numbers from 1 to 8: number 1 being at the extreme right, viewed from behind the group. Thus at a glance, even a casual observer knows what each candidate is saying or doing. The Officer sits at a small table at the focal point of the group, which seems to compel the group to act as a sort of social resonator: a doodle-pad and pencil is on his table.

Officer and Stooge face each other and are edge-on to the semi-circle: seen by all but not distracted by facing the group. The Stooge enters by the door on the right. The PSO sits between the door and number 1. From there, he can conveniently approach the table to speak to the Officer or address the group: or escort the Stooge outside the door and give him additional briefing where necessary.

Observers and visitors—after being introduced—should sit just outside the group in the arc of a larger semi-circle, where their chilling effect is diluted in the group of which they are now almost a part. If there is only one observer, he may sit at the left end of the horse-shoe.

BRIEFING

Only 4 or 5 standardised general briefing points need be made. Cards handed to Officer and Stooge will give them the information they need. These are the sort of points that may usefully be made:—

1 "The object of this session is to get a discussion going on how one should deal with the ordinary human problems which may—and do—occur in any walk of life".

2 "No knowledge of Army procedure is required and ignorance of it will not weigh against you".

3 "We will dramatise these ordinary human problems in 8 short interviews: each interview will take place between one of you representing an Officer who has to deal with the problem and another of you representing the Stooge or "Other Rank" who has asked to see him or is brought before him for a particular reason. Each of you will function once as Officer and once as Stooge".

4 "As Officer, treat the problem in the way you think best: there are no correct answers or procedures but there are a variety of commonsense ways of handling each problem".

5 "The Stooge must really play up to his part: he must identify himself sufficiently with that role to stand up for his own viewpoint: otherwise there will be no clash of wills and no problem for the Officer to solve. The Officer must deal with the problem quickly and expeditiously in the way that seems best and wisest. Three or four minutes should see it through. If you have not finished by then, I may terminate the interview".

6 "Please remember that the prime object of the exercise is to get a discussion going after each interview. When the Officer reads out his card, as he will before the interview begins, may I suggest that you consider how you yourself would handle the problem: then, when the interview is over, you will probably have some comments to contribute". Shifting the emphasis from interview to discussion will make candidates less nervous and more natural in the interview itself.

7 It may be necessary to give the Stooge additional private briefing as one escorts him outside the door while the Officer is reading out the problem on his card to the group: one may stimulate him to play-act his role strongly and consistently or even give him clues about behaviour.

GENERAL ORDER OF PROCEDURE

Officer and Stooge are each handed a card. The Stooge reads his outside the room while the Officer reads his to the group.

E*

While the card informs him as to the Stooge's character and background, he does not know the details or how the Stooge feels about it. After the interview, the Stooge reads his card to the group and then glances at the Officer's. All are now ready for the discussion.

Here are three relatively simple examples:—

Example A

Officer's card: Private Grouse, with a bad disciplinary record, has just returned from 28 days in Detention Barracks. You have decided to see him.

Stooge's card: You have just returned from 28 days' detention. You feel you have had a raw deal and are very embittered. You never wanted to join the Army. You hate everything connected with it and do not intend to do more than will keep you out of further trouble and any more detention. Your OC has sent for you.

The Officer role here to be observed is largely "encouragement" i.e. the ability to help raise the morale of others. The Stooge role here enacted is what the Army colloquially calls "bloody-mindedness" i.e. chronic resentment not amounting to a paranoid reaction. The word "role" is defined on page 131 but we should point out here that it is used in this chapter to cover—*faute de mieux*—two slightly different meanings i.e. the role to be projected, observed and tested in the Officer, and also the role which the Stooge is required deliberately to enact.

Example B

Officer's card: Corporal Goodfellow is too matey with his men. He has been seen in town with them on various occasions. Discipline in his section is falling off. You have sent for him.

Stooge's card: You are a Corporal with many friends in the ranks. You attach a lot of importance to comradeship and do not see why you should discontinue such friendships just because you are a Corporal. Your OC has sent for you.

The Officer role here to be observed is "tact" i.e. the ability to combine firmness with a consideration for the other fellow's self-respect. The Stooge role here is, possibly, some degree of irresponsibility.

Example C

Officer's card: At a recent promotion conference you recommended that Lance-Serjeant Weekly, a rather unsatisfactory and incompetent man, be passed over for promotion. This course was followed and he has now asked to see you.

Stooge's card: You have just been jumped for promotion and think that this is unfair as you feel yourself every bit as good as the chap, a Corporal, promoted ahead of you.

The Officer role is "tact": the Stooge role is that of a discouraged, resentful, somewhat incompetent man.

After the 4-minute interview, the next 6 or 7 minutes of discussion may be conducted in the following 4 phases:—

Phase 1: The group are asked for *spontaneous comments.* Would they handle the problem otherwise? Any comments, criticisms, suggestions?

Phase 2: *Evoked responses* are elicited by the PSO from those who have not yet contributed when and if the discussion abates i.e. "Number 6, what is your feeling about it?" He may ask anyone for comments or put a direct question: and in a group of 8, he may in effect quiz every candidate over the 8 situations: though once a candidate has contributed, he is likely to keep on doing so. The PSO's questions constitute a sort of Group Interview, and should of course avoid suggesting what in his opinion are the correct responses or giving clues as to his own views and individual style of man-management.

Phase 3: The Stooge, if he has not spoken, is asked how he would handle the Officer's problem. One notes his empathic appreciation of his protagonist's role.

Phase 4: The Officer is asked for his reaction to the discussion and whether—in the light of it—he would modify his future handling of such a problem in any way. One notes his capacity for self-assessment, ability to profit from others and possibly his sensitiveness to criticism.

One may ask a second or third pair to handle the original situation if one wishes to exhaust it. There is no reason why the PSO should not improvise new situations or variations: or ask the group to do so. These will constitute a germinating point of experimentation in the test. But standard technique should be used for the query candidates: and the improvised situations should be kept for the end of the session (possibly the last pair) and for the clear-cut candidates.

It is best to start off with a lively spontaneous pair in a lively situation. The one or two query candidates should be brought on half-way through: it is on them one is focussing—without seeming to—throughout the session: then the improvised experimental situations at the end. Obviously, later candidates will conduct a more spontaneous interview: but this must be allowed for.

TIME

With an interview of 4 minutes and an average discussion of 4 to 6 minutes, a 90-minute session should suffice for a group of 8.

PRE-SELECTING OFFICER PROBLEMS AND STOOGE ROLES

Of critical importance to this session is the pre-selection of specific problems and roles that may throw light on the queries raised. Without this, it is of limited value; with it, the results can be—in conjunction with the rest of the testing pattern—profoundly illuminating.

At 10 WOSB it was found convenient for the PSO to cooperate with the Serjeant-Tester or Psychological Officer (who had prepared Pointers for the group) to translate these queries into specific problems and roles. At 5 WOSB, a Key Sheet was devised to assist this translation.

Much work is yet to be done in the devising of a flexible and comprehensive repertoire of test situations. A jumping-off point for such work is provided in this and the next chapter.

Empirically, 28 situations were collected, improved, analysed and classified and seemed to provide sufficient variety from which to select 8 situations for any group. While carefully observing several hundred sessions, one found oneself analysing these 28 situations on one side of a postcard. Along a vertical coordinate one listed them from 1 to 28: along a lateral coordinate one listed —from 1 to 8 or 9—the commoner man-management attitudes and roles that seemed to crop up in the candidates' projection of themselves.

The result of this analysis—after some experimentation— was incorporated into a foolscap Key Sheet: and under the headings of Empathy, Firmness, Encouragement, Tact, etc. were grouped several situations, ranging from easy ones (indicated by a single star) to difficult ones (three starred). Naturally each situation tended to project more than one social role i.e. a Firmness situation might also make demands on the ability to bring others into the picture. The Key Sheet therefore listed both the principal and the auxiliary roles associated with each problem. With its help, problems and Stooge roles could be allocated to every member of the group of 8 in a few moments. One began with the 1 to 3 query candidates, then filled in the rest.

Let us look again at the examples previously given:—

Example A. "The Man Back from the Glasshouse" (two-starred i.e. of moderate difficulty). The principal Officer role is Encouragement, the auxiliary roles Empathy and Firmness. The Stooge role was that of the demoralised delinquent.

Example B. "The Matey Corporal" was classified under Tact (one-starred and the easiest of the 6 situations). The Stooge role was "lack of confidence, poorish morale and slight irresponsibility".

Example C. "The Lance-Serjeant not Promoted" was classified as one of the more difficult of the Tact situations. The Stooge role was that of an inefficient man.

Stooge roles seemed in practice to be especially revealing when he was represented as "bloody-minded" or group-disruptive, irresponsible, selfish, bumptious, or anxious. The bumptious candidate—enacting the role of, say, the "cocky" regimental champion boxer who is throwing his weight about—will make a better Stooge and in so doing help to reveal both his own attitudes and those of his protagonist.

The very tentative classification of commoner Officer problems and Stooge roles given below, derives from a military wartime setting. But while settings vary, the social attitudes required do not: and there should be no difficulty in translating all of these into situations that obtain in any peacetime field of activity.

A TENTATIVE CLASSIFICATION OF OFFICER ROLES

Here we may conveniently consider the word "role" which may be defined as a type of behaviour demanded of individual members of a working group by the job on hand. Different aspects or phases of the job will demand different roles i.e. planning roles, organising roles, social roles, physical roles or the exercise of physical skills, etc. The social roles are concerned with the handling of people in relation to the job, either individually (man-management) or in groups (group-management).

In the implementation of a function (which we define specially on page 141 as a solution or part-solution of the group's problem), many roles may be exercised: and a role may subserve many different functions. In a sense, a role is a collection of skills (physical, mental or social) exercised by an individual and a function is a group-job or part of a group-job.

To illuminate the general with the particular, if the group-job or total function is building a bridge, erecting a pier on the bed of the river will be a part function. That function will demand the exercise of many roles but each of these roles may subserve many different functions.

From the analysis described in the last section, five social roles are here defined and examples given of situations and problems which may be used to elicit and project them. Each role is demanded in some degree of every member of a working team: though to a greater degree on leadership level.

In addition to the five social roles, we will also consider Motivation as meaning here specifically the degree and quality of the self-identification of the candidate with the field of activity for which he is being selected. This is an altitude or predisposition, *not* a social role, but an important one in selection and one which can very conveniently be projected in a session of this kind.

Our six headings then are as follows:—

EMPATHY. The ability to have, and to convey, sympathetic understanding for the emotional reactions and needs of others. It is in a sense a form of emotional participation.

Examples.—handling:—

1 the miserable "rookie" who finds the Army altogether too much for him.
2 the parachutist who has lost his nerve after a near escape.
3 the Commando Serjeant who has just received a telegram that his wife has been ordered to hospital with a surgical emergency: he is a key man, due to leave any moment now on a dangerous but vitally important mission.
4 domestic or personal problems generally.

ENCOURAGEMENT. Knowing when to encourage group-cohesive attitudes in individuals and groups and so to raise individual and group morale: usually by praise, recognition, etc.
Examples—handling:—
1 the parachutist mentioned above.

2 the promising but diffident Lance-corporal who, after two weeks of it, wants to hand in his stripe.

3 the delinquent returned from the "glasshouse", unrepentant and "bloody-minded".

FIRMNESS. The ability to reprimand or take a strong line when it is indicated and to discourage group-disruptive or morale-lowering attitudes in individuals and groups.

Examples—handling:—

1 the bloody-minded "sea-lawyer", a focus of disruption and trouble wherever he goes.

2 the skrimshanker trying to dodge an unpleasant task.

3 the "cocky" regimental boxing champion who is throwing his weight about.

4 any purely disciplinary problems.

TACT. The ability to balance Firmness and Encouragement and to discourage group-disruptive attitudes while maintaining and raising morale: to balance reprimand with face-saving, a "kick in the pants" with a "pat on the back". It may be regarded as a teaching situation in which correction and instruction are fused.

Examples—handling:—

1 the Corporal who lacks confidence and is trying to curry favour with his men by undue familiarity.

2 the efficient NCO with a slight weakness for the ladies who is setting a bad example *vis-a-vis* the ATS personnel in his depot.

3 the Sanitary Corporal, efficient in his humble unattractive job, who could not function as an NCO in any other activity but feels he ought to be promoted.

BRINGING OTHERS INTO THE PICTURE. The ability to relate every member of the group *emotionally* to the group purpose and make him feel he has a part to play in reference to it. This must be distinguished from the ability to relate the group *functionally*—in terms of their capacities and skills—to the group purpose: this capacity for allocation is part of the organising phase of functional ability (p. 31).

It may be noted that of the above five social roles, the first four are *group-binding* roles (they bind the members of the group to each other): the fifth is a *group-relating* role (it relates the group and its members emotionally to the group purpose).

MOTIVATION OR IDENTIFICATION WITH THE FIELD OF ACTIVITY.
It was convenient in wartime to consider identification with
(a) the military *field* generally (b) officer *level* and responsibility, (c) the specific wartime *function* of fighting, as below:—

I. *Identification with the Army generally:* this might be elicited
   in the interview with the miserable recruit who needs
   indoctrination: or as the recruit.

II. *Identification with the Officer role of authority and responsibility:*
    as in handling:—

    1 the man up before his Officer as an eligible "potential
      officer" who should go to WOSB: he refuses how-
      ever to try for a commission for the selfish reason
      that his civilian employers are making his pay up
      and officership will not profit him in any way.
    2 the man who wants to go to WOSB but is quite
      unsuitable: or not yet suitable.

III. *Identification with the combatant role and willingness to fight
     for his country:* as handling:—

    1 the soldier who skrimshanks on the eve of battle.
    2 the technician who—when his Unit is due to go
      overseas—suddenly decides to apply to go to
      WOSB for a commission in another arm of the
      Service: this would of course postpone his over-
      seas posting.

The psychological observer will naturally draw such conclusions as his experience enables him to, about the candidate's
unconscious—as distinct from his conscious—motivation.

A TENTATIVE CLASSIFICATION OF STOOGE ROLES

Though empirical, this list is fairly comprehensive and will
suggest new testing situations for any field. Among the types to
be considered is the Stooge who is:—

1 *anxious* about
   a domestic problems generally
   b separation from home
   c danger in combat
   d responsibility
   e loss of face i.e. at not being promoted, etc.
   f etc., etc.

2 *solitary*, isolate, hypersensitive, unusual in any way, eccentric or even schizoid.

3 of low morale, *discouraged*, bored, "slipping", gets on well with his subordinates but not with his colleagues or superiors, etc.

4 *irresponsible*, babyish, immature, selfish.

5 *inefficient*, slow or slack.

6 *delinquent* i.e. AWOL (absent without leave), the chronic brawler, the mischievous player of practical jokes, etc.

7 rebellious, anti-social, difficult, bloody-minded, *aggressive*, bumptious, conceited, tactless, cannot get on with other people, etc.

8 ambitious or *plus-minded* and wants a more active job: possibly one above his capacity or not now available.

SOME OF THE COMMONER TYPES OF QUERY CANDIDATE

One may not be able to pinpoint and isolate the one particular social role which has been queried: but one can select a situation which will evoke it predominantly. And as, in practice, one is concerned mainly with the 1 to 3 query candidates in the group, additional light can be thrown on the candidate by testing him in the Stooge role and selecting the Officer problem accordingly.

One may usefully note inconsistency or discrepancy between the candidate's projection of himself (1) in the Officer problem (2) the Stooge role, (3) the general discussion and (4) his responses to the PSO's questions. He may profess views in discussion to which he pays little respect in the interview: or honour principles which he finds difficulty in expressing. Here, as elsewhere, discrepancies point to a residual query which determines one's next problem.

One seems to find group-disruptive attitudes more clearly projected in the Stooge role: and the absence of group-cohesive attitudes in the Officer problem. Proneness to anxiety may be revealed in either.

. Some common types of query candidate and the situations likely to be useful are listed below:—

1 Seems *negative and lacking in self-assertiveness*. His problem may require him to reprimand a "bolshy" Stooge: he may be given a timid Stooge role: or a "bloody-

minded" Stooge role—against a strong protagonist—to see if that will rouse him.

2 Seems *irresponsible* and unaware of the implications of authority on officer level. He may be set a "motivation" problem dealing specifically with his identification with the role of authority.

3 Seems *immature*. He may be tested on almost any role, but firmness and empathy are especially convenient.

4 Seems *borderline or limited* through immaturity, inexperience, lack of intelligence or education. Almost any difficult problem, especially those requiring tact.

5 One suspects him of being *carping, discouraging*, disinclined to give praise. Any situation in which he might be expected to give encouragement but could give blame.

6 Seems *thrustful or lacking in empathy*. Any "tact" situation: the situation may be made even more difficult by giving him a strong and difficult Stooge.

Minima in nuce, weak and immature candidates may be tested for firmness: strong, possibly disruptive candidates for empathy, tact, ability to bring others into the picture or—as disruptive Stooges: limited candidates by any problems sufficiently difficult to extend them. The Officer problem reveals the weak, immature or limited: the Stooge role shows up the disruptive.

INTERPRETING THE HUMAN PROBLEMS SESSION

In general, one is concerned not so much with *how* the candidate solves his problem as with what sort of person he reveals himself to be: whether his basic attitude and frame of mind is cohesive or disruptive; and if disruptive, in what respect and which specific social roles he lacks skill in. One proposes to discuss in further detail:—

a the social roles and techniques as exercised in man-management.

b the functional inter-relationships between group, members and task which must be taken into consideration in group-management generally.

SOCIAL ROLES AND TECHNIQUES IN MAN-MANAGEMENT

One cannot hope to classify every possible solution of these "human problems" but one may list some of the commoner ones: as well as the considerations about man-management that come to mind after observing many of these sessions.

In so far as there is an order of approach to the handling of human problems, the four stages to be described are an approximation to it: they are of course not necessarily chronological, but likely to be so.

A first stage is sensing or intuiting the emotional attitudes of others i.e. empathy: and making this empathy explicit i.e. sympathy. To take a lighter social example of the distinction made here (despite etymology) between empathy and sympathy, the man who realises you need a whisky and soda has empathy: if he offers you one, he has sympathy. Sympathy is the implementation of one's empathy. In the "Human Problems" interview, even a statement indicating that one understands will constitute a preliminary act of sympathy.

Associated with this first stage is the handling of grievances and anxiety. Where there is an element of grievance, the emotional charge of suppressed aggression must be "drained": the grievant must be *unburdened* of his load before any constructive approach to his problem can be attempted. The same "drainage" or unburdening is necessary with anxiety or fear. In short, any emotional charge of anxiety, fear or aggression—overt or partly suppressed—must be revealed and allowed to discharge itself before a sufficiently warm contact can be established to permit of tackling the man's problem.

After seeing a man's viewpoint and making it clear that one does, the second stage is to help him re-establish "face" if he has lost it. Understanding and sympathy in themselves will help: but it may be necessary in addition to encourage him: to give specific reasons why he should have a better opinion of himself, in certain respects, than he now has.

A third stage is to help him see the viewpoint and purpose of the group: to relate him to the Law of the Total Situation. This one does by (a) discouraging group-disruptive attitudes (b) encouraging group-cohesive attitudes and explaining why, in terms of the LOTS.

Encouraging group-cohesive attitudes in a man is of course not the same as encouraging his ego (as in the second stage). The latter is an attempt to unify the man and the conflicting parts of his personality: the former is an attempt to unify the group by binding him to it. The one is an aspect of *man-manage-*

ment i.e. unifying and organising the man (a sort of minor psychotherapy): the other is an aspect of *group-management* i.e. unifying and organising the group.

The discouraging of group-disruptive attitudes may entail firmness and this should be preceded by encouragement: as in the age-old Oriental wisdom of preceding correction by "face-saving". A possible exception is in crisis or emergency or with repeated disruptive behaviour where a sharp immediate reproof may precede any later attempt to raise morale. The situations where one may legitimately and usefully *allow* oneself to lose one's temper can probably be handled only by those with very considerable experience: and *they* are least likely to allow such situations to arise. They too may feel the occasional need to vent frustrated emotions, but no doubt will relate it to tactical needs.

Firmness of this kind bears little relationship to the dominance and aggressiveness which some psychologists—especially in USA—seem to regard as closely correlated with leadership. One's experience is that dominant or aggressive people are rightfully resented by the group: their effectiveness is diminished rather than enhanced thereby: if leadership accrues, it is despite this handicap.

If there is a relationship between aggressive dominance and leadership, it might more easily be an inverse one. In so far as aggression has been disciplined and harnessed effectively, it is unlikely to become apparent as aggressiveness—or even dominance. If Ascendance-submissiveness tests measure anything, they measure a man's free floating unharnessed aggression and potential group-disruptive capacity rather than his capacity to influence people firmly but tactfully. Moreover misplaced aggression is unlikely to lead to that constructive use of conflict discussed below which is the basis of all high-level leadership.

Incidentally, the firmness of the ordinary simple command —as in drill, where no rebuke or correction is implied—is not so much firmness as audibility and precision of speech, an aspect of verbal expression: which not all drill Serjeants may realise.

The fourth and last stage in man-management is to bring the man right into the picture and commit him to some sort of fruitful participation in the group's activities. If (a) he is a *participant* and *his participation has seemed* to him (b) *interesting* (c) *of value* and (d) *appreciated*, he will be provided with the best

positive incentive to maintain and develop it. Indeed the whole
vexed question of positive incentives may boil down to this.
When these four criteria are present, it is unlikely that he will
resent tactful and constructive criticism of his shortcomings.

In the Human Problems Session, this fruitful participation
can necessarily amount only to his contributing plans or suggestions likely to be accepted by others as an improvement. The
Officer may induce this participation by knowing when and how
to invite, accept, use and give credit for suggestions: by "consulting the Stooge" as to what he thinks has gone wrong, how it
might have been prevented, what can be done to remedy it.

The situation is revealed to the Stooge as a problem to be
solved by Officer and Stooge in cooperation. From the Officer's
viewpoint, in so far as he is senior in leadership, it becomes a
teaching situation: for he has necessarily more to contribute to
that cooperation: especially so when dealing with the inefficient
and delinquent.

If the Stooge's suggestions do not include effective ones,
others may be fed to him; including that which seems wisest.
One might use the analogy—not really a just one—of the con-
jurer "forcing a card". The object is to lead him to feel the
suggestion is his or that he has contributed to it. In short, he
should be invited to participate and induced to accept that
invitation.

A TENTATIVE FORMULATION OF GROUP-MANAGEMENT PRINCIPLES

After one's first draft of this book, one came across the contributions of Mary Parker Follett in her collected papers "Dynamic
Administration" (edited by L. Urwick and H. C. Metcalf,
London 1941). This remarkable woman, over a period of 25
years, formulated ideas well in advance of her time.

One's own reactions to her suggestions—which WOSB
experience of experimental groups seems to confirm—lead one
to suggest a very tentative formulation of the relationships
between a group, its activities and the Law of the Total Situation
(LOTS) i.e. the total problem which confronts it. A formulation
which relates the concepts of leadership, function, authority,
control, orders, commands, directives etc.: and may lead to
preciser concepts of leadership function and functional roles.

It may be expressed in this way:—

A conflict or crisis is precipitated by discrepancies and differences: discrepancies between effort and achievement or revealed in the process of trial or error: differences of opinion, of aims and interests, of types of personality or ability.

Such a conflict indicates always:—

a that a new problem—a new query—has arisen:

b that a solution of the problem on a higher level of function is indicated: higher in that it must successfully integrate what previously has been uncoordinated and seemingly irreconcilable.

c that there is need for a referral back to the LOTS and for its reconsideration in the perspective of the changing situation.

The total situation is necessarily a situation in flux; and conflict indicates a major change which the group has either failed to anticipate or perceive or had time to adapt to. Only by perceiving this change clearly and objectively and by formulating the real problem and the real query as they now are can one hope to find the real answer and effective solution.

Those whose attitude is group-cohesive will aim to use conflict constructively to bind the group on a higher level of function: by presenting it as a query requiring an answer. They will realise the need of clustering points of essential difference and essential similarity: of spot-lighting the former in order to focus collective enquiry on them: of correlating at every point general aims with specific efforts.

Those whose attitude is group-disruptive will see conflict not as a pointer to the need for integration on a higher level but as a threat and challenge to the dominance of specific individuals or sub-groups. They will see it emotionally rather than objectively: their emotional pre-disposition is to fighting it out rather than to thinking it out: their influence is towards disrupting the group into sections or sides, towards schism and wastage of group power.

Formulating the real query and finding its solution and answer and thus re-constituting a new Gestalt, a new LOTS, constitutes the "planning" phase of functional ability discussed on page 31. Differentiating the solution into its component functions and allocating these in terms of people, roles, material, space and time constitutes the "organising" phase there discussed. The actual execution of each component function constitutes the phase of "practical execution."

Corresponding to the solution of the problem and determined by it is the *Imperative* to the group and to every member of it: and that Imperative may be differentiated into its component Sub-imperatives or *Orders* either to each member of the group or in relation to individual functions. The Imperative corresponds to the total pattern of functions and their inter-relationship as implied in the solution: and is the sanction and demand for their execution. The Orders correspond to individual component functions and are the sanction and demand for their execution in the organising phase and for the various roles needed in their execution.

In the phase of "practical execution", Orders will be made explicit either in written *Directives*, spoken *Commands* or practical *Demonstrations or Example*. The Order not only determines the function of every member of the group but also the *Authority* and *Responsibility* that goes with it.

In this sense, the right and obligation to exercise authority, the obligation to exercise it responsibly and the extent of that authority and responsibility are determined by the function: which in turn derives from the Order, the general Imperative and ultimately the LOTS. Where this changes and is re-constituted—as it will in the course of its natural flux or where major conflict has compelled it—it will determine anew the whole pattern of functions.

Power may be considered as the potential energy of a group—in relation to a specific group task—deriving from the coordination of all the individual functional abilities in the group.

Control may be regarded as the limiting effect of individual functions on each other, and of total function on part functions: perhaps as the equilibrium established between cohesive and disruptive influences: techniques for its implementation laterally and vertically are not discussed here.

From this tentative formulation—intended only to stimulate observation and analysis of small experimental groups or of larger groups in the community—three interesting suggestions emerge:—

    1 It does suggest that conflict may be viewed constructively by regarding it as a query which demands a solution on a higher level. Mary Parker Follett comments cogently

on this point. She points out that where one side dominates and wins the issue, the other side is dissatisfied:
in compromise, neither side is completely satisfied: both
domination and compromise are inferior to a solution
which destroys the schism, unifies the group and in so
doing necessarily produces a higher level of efficiency.

2 By deriving primary authority from the solution to the
group-problem (LOTS) and secondary authority from
its component functions, real leadership is seen to be
collectively vested. Emphasis is taken from the leadership of one man and placed on a common group purpose
which all must serve. "Institutional" leadership (by
virtue of rank) is not leadership at all: it is the exercise
of vested authority. If that vested authority corresponds
with the function actually exercised, there is real leadership: but it may not.

3 It questions decisively the concept that a Command or
Directive automatically carries the right to blind obedi-
ence. If we assume that the Command is an expression
of the Order which derives from the LOTS, then the
officer or leader who gives a Command which does not
express the true Order must be regarded as responsible
for his incapacity to interpret the Order or translate it
into the appropriate Command. Bad Commands will
ultimately disrupt the group as well as nullify its achievement: and though the time element may on occasion
demand snap Commands though imperfect and more
liable to error, on the whole some machinery is desirable
for referring bad Commands—and their givers—back to
their ultimate justification—the LOTS.

To summarise briefly:—

Conflict or crisis—viewed constructively—reveals a problem
which may be formulated as a query. To resolve the query, true
leadership will refer back to the total situation: and a clarification
and re-statement of the LOTS determines the Imperative or
sanction to the group with its Sub-imperatives or Orders which
authorise and initiate individual functions in the group. These
LOTS-determined functions (a) carry with them the real organic
authority required to implement them—and no more, (b) they
determine and limit the extent of the responsibility for implementing them.

As the LOTS is necessarily in flux in adaptation to the changing problem, so everything determined by it must be capable of a corresponding change. The recurrence of over-frequent conflicts or of conflicts amounting to crisis will suggest that the machinery of group procedures for correlating all of these is insufficiently flexible.

SOME DIFFICULTIES AND OBJECTIONS

It has been objected—usually by those who have not had an opportunity of seeing the session adequately conducted or have not appreciated its nature and rationale—that:—

    a it is unfair to the immature candidate with little worldly experience:

    b it favours the "actor":

    c it is difficult and unreliable.

Let us discuss these in order.

IS THE SESSION UNFAIR TO THE IMMATURE?

This is based on the serious misconception that Army knowledge and experience in man-management are the all-important factors in a good performance.

In this task is contained (a) a functional component i.e. dealing effectively with the situation, (b) a social component i.e. manifesting certain social abilities which may be summed up as group-cohesiveness. This session is mainly concerned with the latter and with inducing the candidate to reveal in behaviour whether his trend is cohesive or disruptive.

The less his experience of man-management—and consequently the less he knows of the conventional stereotypic solutions—the more he will be compelled to fall back on his own natural attitudes. Not knowing what to do, he is compelled to improvise with whatever spontaneity he has got. Interpreted and conducted in this way, the session is possibly more useful—so one would contend—with the young and inexperienced than with the worldly-wise.

But even if the more experienced candidate reveals the extent of his experience rather than his basic social attitudes—and one does not agree that with the technique here described, this is necessarily so—even this revelation of his experience constitutes useful information about him. But there is, of course, every reason why one should note both his experience *and* his social attitudes.

IS THE "ACTOR" AT AN ADVANTAGE?

It has been objected that the Officer may consciously dis-simulate and play a part not natural to him.

In the first instance, he would need to know what role to enact. To realise that certain social attitudes are considered to be wise and to merit approval is—if they are actually cohesive attitudes—perhaps a step towards social maturity. "To be aware of" is perhaps not so good as "to be identified with" but it is one developmental phase ahead of "to be completely unaware of".

If one visualises the pattern of WOSB testing, one will realise that many factors tend to prevent self-conscious acting: apart from the fact that the specific aim of the testing technique is to induce spontaneity. Such factors as the following: in a 4-minute stress interview, the candidate has no more than 30 seconds to peruse his card and prepare his campaign: the details and Stooge attitudes are not known to him: both protagonists are pre-selected, and the Stooge specially briefed, to create a clash of wills: observer and watching group by now know quite a lot about him and would be quick to sense insincerity: the candidate too is well aware of this. A point of incidental interest is that the would-be dissimulator is the first to suspect insincerity in others, and may reveal in discussion his readiness to suspect the worst.

It has been objected that as the Stooge is specially enjoined to play-act his role, it is not quite fair to devaluate him because he has followed his instructions faithfully. Experience suggests that most men have difficulty in enacting roles with which they have nothing in common. In one's own experience of this session, there seemed to be no difficulty in differentiating between acting ability and emotional predilection for a role: the "actor" was rare and never seemed reluctant to reveal himself.

IS THE SESSION TOO DIFFICULT AND UNRELIABLE?

This critical question cannot be evaded and compels us to face the fact that no projective session can be adequately or use-fully conducted without psychological help and supervision. Conducted without appreciation of its purpose—or skill and experience in its interpretation—it is useless, time-consuming and misleading.

As projective techniques seem to be the germinating point of technical development in personality evaluation (apart from intelligence tests and biographical questionnaires, there is little in WOSB testing that has not a projective element), psychological cooperation and technical supervision cannot be dispensed with if the unchecked, uncurbed "hunch" is not to decide the fate of men. It is unfair to expect those who are not psychologically trained to bear the full burden of a projective session. It is however only fair—to candidates who are being selected for roles of responsibility and leadership and whose careers depend on the choice—that their selectors should possess the minimal ability and flair that will enable them, after adequate training, to work in a team whose purpose is primarily psychological.

The real answer to this objection seems to be that a session of this type should be conducted jointly by a PSO and a member of the psychological team. A procedure along these lines was carried out at 10 WOSB and 5 WOSB: the Serjeant-tester collaborated with the PSO in pre-selecting problems and roles: while the psychiatrist and psychological officer were allowed to participate in the actual session.

A RESUME OF BASIC PRINCIPLES

1 The Human Problems Session is a "selective oral projection" session whose purpose is to help resolve queries about candidates —in respect of their group-cohesiveness and aptitude in specific social roles—which have been raised either at the Query Conference (from observation of the Basic Series) or from a Personality Pointer.

2 In 8 short stress interviews (each followed by group discussion), each candidate acts once as an Officer required to solve a human problem of the type that may arise in his work: and once as the Stooge who is required to enact a protagonist role. Each knows only part of the facts and the situation is so planned that a stress factor is implicit and a clash of wills inevitable.

3 In briefing the session, more emphasis is placed on the discussion than on the interviews which provoke it: in the hope that the tension and nervousness of Stooge and Officer will be diminished and their spontaneity and self-revelation increased.

4 A projection of each candidate's social attitudes is obtained from (a) his solving of the Officer problem, (b) his playing of the Stooge role, (c) his participation in the discussion, and possibly (d) his responses to the PSO's questions. The impression gained from this combined fourfold projection is analysed and

evaluated and considered in the light of *all* the available evidence up to date.

5 The Officer problem and Stooge role are pre-selected for each candidate; preferably by the PSO in collaboration with a member of the psychological team i.e. the Serjeant-tester who has analysed the Personality Pointers for that group. Special attention is paid to the 1 to 3 query candidates. While the solution of the Officer problem is usually the more revealing part of the interview, the interview may be so planned as to throw light on the Stooge rather than the Officer.

6 The Officer is judged not so much by his solution of the problem (which may be influenced by experience or knowledge) as by his manner of handling it: and specifically by his ability to cope flexibly, spontaneously, group-cohesively and with appropriate improvisations with the changing dynamics of the social situation. The Officer problem is especially helpful in revealing the absence of group-cohesive attitudes.

7 It is hoped that the Stooge, in playing his role, will project —as distinct from his acting ability—certain attitudes basic to his nature that have been queried. The Stooge role is especially helpful in revealing group-disruptive attitudes.

8 The group—in semicircle or horseshoe—acts:—

a partly as a social resonator to intensify the Officer-Stooge clash:

b partly as an interacting audience whose empathic reactions produce a progressive rise in the emotional temperature of the group with a corresponding increase in animation, spontaneity and naturalness in projecting emotional attitudes:

c partly to provide the PSO with the opportunity for a group interview in which he may interrogate and purposefully stimulate certain candidates.

9 If the session is carried out reasonably well, the linkage of eight interviews by discussion results in a field of increasingly more fluid and intensified reactions in which all are participating directly or empathically. Anyone not participating may be directly invited to do so.

10 One must keep in mind:—

a by the time one comes to this session, one already knows a great deal about each candidate.

b one is mainly interested in the 1 to 3 query candidates: for the others the session is largely confirmatory.

c the session is but one item in the entire observational field to be related to the rest of the evidence.

d as the evidence is of a projective nature, it must be carefully evaluated and interpreted as such: for this, psychological help and supervision is necessary.

11 One's own predilection is for making the Human Problems Session the last and Final Exercise to constitute Phase 3 and to be observed by the entire observer team (with a good technique, the presence of the team will enhance rather than chill the session). Each candidate would be seen "in the round" for the last time and ultimate queries about his social personality resolved.

12 Much work remains to be done on Officer problems, Stooge roles and man-management techniques generally. This type of session—which is similar to the "psychodramatic" techniques used by Moreno for therapeutic purposes—is likely to prove of increasing value for training, educative and therapeutic purposes as well as for selective and diagnostic purposes.

For the training of man-management and group-management roles on all levels of leadership, it could be especially useful. Just as a schoolboy may now be taught to use the calculus—once only possible to the advanced mathematician—so it should be possible to teach the better approaches to man-management and group-management to the lance-corporal, the charge-hand, the junior leader and to those vested with high authority but not necessarily experienced in its use.

CHAPTER XIV

THE PROJECTIVE PSYCHIATRIC INTERVIEW

ITS PURPOSE AND RELATIONSHIP TO THE REST OF BOARD
PROCEDURE . . . . page 148

THREE FUNCTIONS OF THE SELECTION INTERVIEW CON-
SIDERED AS A TEST PROCEDURE . . . . . ,, 150

   I CHECKING UP ON THE CANDIDATE'S LEVEL . . . . ,, 150

   II PROJECTING THE CANDIDATE'S BIA IN ORDER TO ESTIMATE HIS
      GROUP-COHESIVENESS . . . . ,, 154

      A—THE CONTROL OF STRESS IN THE PROJECTIVE INTERVIEW . . ,, 154

      B—ANALYSING THE CANDIDATE'S REACTION TO YOU: HIS BIA AND BFA ,, 158
         The Mature Co-operative or Objective Personality (MATCOP)
         The Immature-aggressive Personality (IMAG)
         The Immature-dependent Personality (IMDEP)

      C—ANALYSING—AND ALLOWING FOR—YOUR REACTION TO THE
         CANDIDATE: THE COUNTER-TRANSFERENCE . . . ,, 162

      D—FIVE SIGNS OF A "ROBUST SANITY" . . . . . ,, 163
         WARMTH of Feeling
         SPONTANEITY of Expressive Behaviour
         OBJECTIVITY of Social Thinking
         CO-OPERATIVENESS of Social Behaviour
         COMMENSURATE EFFECTIVENESS of Total—including
          Functional-Behaviour

      E—A 3-POINT RATING OF SOCIAL MATURITY . . . . ,, 178

   III EVALUATING THE CANDIDATE'S STABILITY . . . . ,, 181

THE ORDER OF PROCEDURE . . . . ,, 186

OPTIMUM CONDITIONS FOR THE INTERVIEW . . . ,, 192

REPORTAGE . . . . ,, 194

ITS PURPOSE AND RELATIONSHIP TO
THE REST OF BOARD PROCEDURE

The medical psychologist, come to selection, soon realises how different the selection interview is from the therapeutic: the patient strongly wishes to unburden himself, the candidate may equally strongly wish to keep his true personality to himself: he is out not so much to reveal as to "sell" himself.

WOSB procedure may be regarded as a multiple sandwich of alternate tests and screenings. The purpose of a test is to find the best answer one can to the most specific, most clearly formulated question one can put (the question may derive from a previous screening): the purpose of a screening or filter is to sift and compare answers to a test or tests: to note points of agreement and discrepancy: and, if there is not sufficient agreement, to formulate residual queries for another testing phase. Points of disagreement in the results of different tests or in the evaluation of the same test by different observers will constitute provisional queries for a new testing phase: points of agreement will constitute provisional hypotheses to be verified, confirmed or rebutted.

The screen or filter tends to hold in its meshes for further investigation the inconsistencies, discrepancies and incomplete items and to allow through, the agreements and consistencies. It is the alternation of testing and screening phases in the WOSB 3-phase sandwich that so considerably multiplies its effectiveness.

In brief, a test formulates the questions and gets the answers: a screen *sifts* the answers and may leave residual queries. The preliminary paper work, for example constitutes a test of the candidate, the Personality Pointer derived from it is a screening of his responses: the Basic Series is a battery of tests, the Query Conference its screening: the PSO battery and interviews are test procedures, the Interim Grading their screening: the Final Exercise is a test: the Judgement Test is partly a test of group reactions, partly a screening of discrepant from shared opinions: the Final Board is the ultimate and most elaborate screening around whose points of agreement the final decision crystallises.

As a test procedure the selection interview has at least three functions to perform:—

1 *to check up on* the candidate's *potential functional level* in relation to the job's requirements;

2 *to "project"* the quality of his characteristic social behaviour and *group-cohesiveness;*

3 *to evaluate*—from a consideration of (1) and (2) and other relevant factors, such as morale and health, his *likely stability in relation to the* level and field of the *job.*

Because the candidate has more incentive to display a façade than to unburden himself, the cathartic interview of therapy must give way to a projective technique which aims to induce behaviour as spontaneously characteristic as possible. One might usefully emphasise the distinction by calling the selection interview a "projective psychiatric interview".

For the WOSB psychiatrist, the projective interview is the heart of the sandwich: all preceding tests are screened to raise the queries it is to answer; and to formulate the hypotheses it is to confirm or rebut. The better that screening, the profounder the investigation possible.

The answers obtained and the unresolved discrepancies constitute hypotheses and queries for the next phase. The interview links up with what goes before and comes after: there may also be a lateral linkage with the tests and other interviews of phase 2. In short, the selection interview is not only a projective interview: it is also a related interview: one item in selection board procedure.

While the Psychiatrist should screen all candidates, he cannot efficiently interview all in a 3-day Board if there are more than a dozen. The system of priorities described in Chapter XI by which he interviews about one in four constitutes a useful screening for interview. Another useful screening became possible when one did one's interviewing in two sessions on subsequent days with an intervening testing period. Out of, say, a dozen queries or referrals, one interviewed the four most obviously complex in the first session: by the time the second session came round, the picture had usually clarified itself about 3 or 4 of the remainder: leaving the rest for more intensive investigation. A third screening effect can be obtained by interviewing a candidate after the Final Exercise or the Judgement Test: when he has shown doubtful traits comparatively late or when the discrepant opinions of observers have not by then been "ironed out" and another opinion is desirable.

THREE FUNCTIONS OF THE SELECTION INTERVIEW CONSIDERED AS A TEST PROCEDURE

I—CHECKING UP ON THE CANDIDATE'S LEVEL

Sources of Information

Data from which to evaluate level may be obtained from:—

1 the first and second screening elements of the Pointer: also from the Interests Questionnaire in the third element in so far as it indicates range and intensity of interests relevant to the job;

2 such samples of planning as may be thrown up by the Basic Series and other tests i.e. Planning Project, Command Situations, etc.; negative evidence however may not be conclusive:

3 such further information as can be obtained in the interview: that the quality of a man's thinking can sometimes be sampled is suggested below.

Potential, Actual, Aspired and Self-estimated Levels in Relation to the Level Required by the Job

Certain aspects of a man's level may usefully be kept in mind:—

1 his *Potential* functional *Level* (PL) as indicated by intelligence, education, experience, range and intensity of interests, etc.; *especially the first two:*

2 his *Actual* present *Level* (AL) as indicated by his past achievement, recent opinions on his work, the Basic Series and other tests, the interview:

3 his *Self-estimated Level* (SEL) i.e. how he rates his own capacity (its objectivity is important in so far as it influences LA below):

4 his *Level of Aspiration* (LA) and the degree to which this relates to (1) and (5):

5 the *Required Level* (RL) as demanded by the job and as determined by a job-analysis or other estimate.

One feels tempted to add, his *Opted Level* i.e. the level within his own range of function (it may be relatively high or low) on which he elects to work.

The inter-relationships between these levels are important; gaps, lags and discrepancies may automatically raise queries or explain ineffectiveness or instability. To clarify them, one must ask several questions.

Has He Got the Potential or Actual Ability?

Has he got "what it takes"? Is the ratio between AL and RL adequate? If the ratio between PL and RL is adequate, is he developing the former so as to increase his AL?

F

What struck one forcibly in officer selection—one had not realised it to the same extent in therapeutic work because intelligence ratings were not so freely available—was the number of men whose maladjustments were due to attempting tasks well above their optimum level: driven either by an inner urge to compensate for some insecurity or by parents compensating for their own frustrations. However, the number of those whose maladjustment derives from unusually high ability with insufficient opportunity or outlet is probably considerably more.

One may ask, what should the RL be?

WOSB experience (p. 57) suggests that average officer level is about OIR 6–7/ES 31 or 32 i.e. an intelligence level ranging roughly between the 90th to the 98th percentile in the general population, with about School Certificate standard of education. For technical arms, probably a slightly higher average is optimal i.e. OIR 8/ES 22 (from the 98th percentile upward, with Higher School Certificate standard of education).

This RL is probably a sufficiently good approximation for those to be trained for managerial, professional or administrative function or leadership in any field. A higher level may increase stability or counterbalance a defect. A lower level—if the discrepancy is moderate—may be counterbalanced by unusually good group-cohesiveness, strong physical drive, a high LA combined with an objective estimate of one's ability in relation to the task one has set oneself. Deciding to what extent one should encourage, permit or discourage a powerful compensatory urge is indeed a delicate and important responsibility.

To What Effect Has He Been Using His Ability?

Assuming in the first instance he has got "what it takes", what use has he been making of his ability and to what extent is it continuing to grow?

Why has this candidate, whose intelligence is high and whose education has been good, failed to pass his exams? Or, having passed them, why has he failed to do work commensurate with his true ability? Is there a difficult home? Some external obstacle or internal inhibition?

Is there a material lag between his AL and PL and is his AL on the rise or fall? His PL, his AL and its present direction should between them—against a background of the known data—plot a curve to indicate at any rate his near future.

Is His Level of Aspiration Adequate and Objective?

The next two questions are:—

1 Is he determined to use his ability on leadership level i.e. is his LA high enough? Or is he not sufficiently identified with responsibility on that level?

2 Is his LA objectively related to his true abilities or PA?

In so far as his SEL is objective and mature and he realises his strengths as well as his weaknesses, his LA will be sufficiently high to implement his abilities on leadership level.

In so far as his attitude is immature and ambivalent, he will tend to overtax or undertax his capacity: to aim unduly high or unduly low; to overcompensate wildly for a profound sense of insecurity or lapse into demoralisation and make little or no attempt to develop to his own natural level (laziness is likely to be a symptom of such demoralisation). Such an attitude points in the direction of maladjustment or instability.

Sampling the Quality of a Man's Thinking

One's own feeling is that the interview can often be used to sample the quality of a man's thinking. It is not necessarily easy but with increasing experience, one feels, possible. One found oneself considering this quality empirically and clinically in terms of three dimensions i.e. height, width and depth.

Height is the acuity as indicated by intelligence level on testing. *Width* is the range of interests, ideas and topics over which—by virtue of sufficient interest and knowledge—a man is able to exercise this acuity. *Depth* (the most difficult concept and the most difficult dimension to evaluate) is his capacity for fresh, spontaneous, original and independent thinking on subjects not familiar to him: his ability to manipulate abstract concepts freely and constructively and even creatively rather than to reproduce what he or others have said or thought before.

Depth is not entirely a function of *Height* and *Width* though it is likely to be strongly related to them. Only exceptional candidates will show it to marked degree: yet some promise of it should be present in any one whose intelligence and education brings him within the range of potential leadership.

At one end of the scale is the "three-dimensional" thinker, who can take a topic new to him, think round it frankly and spontaneously and perhaps arrive—in the actual interview—at conclusions new and original to him. At the other end is the "cliché" or "gramophone record" mind whose stereotypy in thinking may derive from immaturity, fear, escape into rigid convention, inhibition of natural spontaneity or—an intelligence not sufficiently high.

II—Projecting the Candidate's BIA in Order to Estimate His Group-cohesiveness

The projective function of the interview is the most important —especially when selecting potential leaders—and may be considered under four headings:—

a One must so control the stress implicit in the interview (which is a test) as to get a spontaneous and characteristic sample of the candidate's social behaviour.

b One must specifically note and analyse the candidate's reaction and attitude to oneself (his emotional transference): this should contain a sample of his BIA (basic interpersonal attitudes) and may give a clue—in conjunction with his history— to his prototypic BFA (basic family attitudes) i.e. the pattern of his early object-relationships and attitudes to the parental figures.

c One must analyse—and allow for—one's own spontaneous emotional reactions to the candidate in the course of the interview i.e. one's counter-transference.

d One may—in extension of (*b*)—relate the candidate's attitude and behaviour in interview to certain criteria of superior personality and adjustment, derived from clinical experience or investigation. This topic will be developed in detail.

A—THE CONTROL OF STRESS IN THE PROJECTIVE INTERVIEW

No selection interview can be entirely free from the stress of being weighed in the balance—on trial and on test—with the possibility of being found wanting. Some stress is implicit in the mere fact of being interviewed for an opportunity which may raise the level of one's life. Nor does one wish to remove all of this, even if one could: indeed the candidate's handling of this anxious situation may give important clues to his maturity, morale and stability.

But ordinarily one will reduce the stress, de-tense the candidate and put him at his ease. On page 61, it was suggested that a spontaneous reaction may be induced by the contrasting methods of putting a man at his ease or jolting him suddenly: by diminishing the tension, or suddenly increasing it. The one lulls his inhibitions, the other momentarily disarms or paralyses them.

Because the candidate often cannot or will not cooperate with the frankness one may legitimately expect in an aspirant to opportunity, authority and responsibility, the handling of the interview may have to vary from a passive yielding to the candidate's personality in which he is lulled and de-tensed: through a less passive yielding in which he is given the reins and allowed to take charge of the interview and to control its stresses and tensions himself: to an active attack or jolt which compels him to react immediately and therefore with some degree of spontaneity. Because of this need to control the stress dynamics of the interview, interviewing cannot be otherwise than a sensitive and flexible art.

One found it useful to think of the strategy of stress control in the interview in terms of Judo (the Zen philosophy of ju-jitsu, whose practice and principles had interested me): that is to say, first in terms of a purposive alternation of yielding and attack, of diminishing and increasing stress: then later, in a transcending of both phases in a unified attitude which will be discussed below. In terms of these analogies, we will consider three techniques which we will call the "Lull", the "Jolt" and the "Follow" techniques.

The "Lull" Technique

With this technique, one gives the candidate every help and reassurance, allows and encourages him to linger on his happier more successful experiences, on his virtues and stronger points: allows him to skim—if he so wishes—his weaker more tender points.

With two types of candidate, this is especially useful:—

1 the timid, shy, socially inhibited candidate who may not otherwise emerge from his shell:

2 the expansive psychopath, the overactive hypomanic, the grossly thrusting over-compensator who is "shooting a line": by yielding to the impetus of his compensatory thrust, inflated ego and aggressive self-salesmanship, he will unbalance himself and sprawl before you in all his obvious instability.

The "Jolt" Technique

This must be used with much discretion and always "sealed off". No candidate should leave the interview feeling hurt or with diminished confidence: it should, if at all possible, be of help to him. Even the completely bogus—who are rare—should be merely discarded: there may be a place for moral exhortation but *not* in the selection interview. The goodwill which derives from the doctor-patient relationship must never be sacrificed or abused nor its function exceeded.

One may use:—

 a A lingering on points of stress, friction or maladjustment in the candidate's history; on awkward discrepancies from the Pointers; on the candidate's behaviour at the impasses of the Basic Series.

 b A sudden challenge by critical provocative questions.

 c A most powerful "jolt" technique is the "silent pause" described by Dr. J. Rickman as a test of the candidate's capacity to tolerate the tensions raised within himself by the psychiatric interview. The stressfulness of this pause—which consists of the interviewer saying absolutely nothing for a full minute or two—when introduced at suitable points may force a revealing admission of personality or a sample of the candidate's habitual reaction to anxiety i.e. over-conciliation, self-depreciation, facetiousness, aggressiveness, etc.

 d Any "jolt" technique may be reinforced by altering the tempo of the interview suddenly and often: by alternating the pleasant and the stressful: by a rapid glissando from yielding to attack, from lull to jolt.

The "jolt" may be useful with:—

 a The very inhibited, "shut-in", slightly negativistic, apathetic or any who do not react to the "lull" technique.

 b Some who are difficult, resentful, refractory or brusque. Where the brusqueness derives from a difficult son-father relationship which has been activated in the interview, the candidate may sometimes be jolted by counter-brusqueness into a more spontaneous frankness.

 c Those one has reason to consider untruthful, deceitful or "bogus": the "sealing" will require tact.

 d The over-conciliatory and over-suggestible in whom one

suspects a markedly ambivalent attitude: with considerable aggression near the surface which may be provoked into emergence.

The "Follow" Technique

With increasing volume of experience and a new emergent level of skill, one should find oneself adopting what one might call a "follow" technique in which one gives the candidate the reins but lulls and jolts—slightly—as occasion demands.

To continue the Judo analogy. In the phasic alternation of yielding and attack which constitutes Judo wrestling, it is at first necessary to stress—for the beginner—the importance of yielding: for the reason that instinct favours attack rather than the more economical, more effective co-ordination of yielding *and* attack. At a later stage, the principle of "Wu-wei" is introduced. Wu-wei derives from Zen philosophy—mothered by Buddhism and fathered by Taoism—which inspired the Golden Age of T'ang and Sung Chinese Art, most Japanese art and poetry and many allied cultural and practical arts i.e. the Sumiye genre of black and white painting, the Tea Ceremony, Noh Plays, flower and landscape arrangement, fencing, Judo wrestling, etc.

In Judo, Wu-wei (which may be translated as "action in inaction", "effortless action", "no interference", "no pressing" or "no strain") expresses itself in a principle which transcends passive yielding and active attack but includes—and intensifies—both in a fluid process of feeling oneself "at one with" one's opponent: one follows his thrusts or his retreats spontaneously with a sort of counter-yielding to his push and counter-attack to his yielding. At this stage the wrestler is not aware of himself either yielding or attacking: each phase flows naturally into the other, unpunctuated by perceptible jump or jerk, without a hairsbreadth between either.

Similarly in the interview, the first tendency of the inexperienced interviewer is to be active, to thrust forward, to make the aggressive attack of the direct—often brutally direct—question. Though useful as an occasional and deliberate "jolt" technique, as an exclusive technique it is deadly, and destructive of every germ of spontaneity. The psychotherapist has long learnt to let his patient take the initiative and to yield sensitively and sympathetically to the thrust of his personality. But this yielding phase must very definitely be learnt.

The optimum technique is achieved when, for the most part, one follows the interviewee but lets him have his own way: one neither denies nor affirms but gives, goes with, is "at one with". One does not so much yield or attack, lull or jolt, as follow his yieldings and his thrusts. One may push slightly when he is about to stop yielding and yield slightly before he has stopped pushing: ordinarily neither push nor yield is clearly noted as such: but there are times when—to test or unbalance him—one yields a little more or pushes a little more.

In short, the best way to control the stress element implicit in the selection interview is by a "follow" technique in which one lets the candidate follow his own course but interjects—where experience suggests it will aid the candidate to project himself— a lulling influence or a jolting impetus. In a flexibly following technique of this kind, one seals the stressful points automatically as one goes along. Where a powerful isolated jolt is used for a special reason it must just as deliberately be sealed and the manner of doing this is discussed later.

B—ANALYSING THE CANDIDATE'S REACTION TO YOU:
HIS BIA AND BFA

If as medical psychologist one is to make a predictive estimate of a candidate's likely behaviour and stability, one must study him not only in social area but also in depth, not only his social reactions in the group but also their determinants: their socio-dynamics as well as their psychodynamics, his BIA as well as his BFA. This one ordinarily does in the psychiatric interview.

The sociodynamic or area aspect was touched on in Chapter x in considering three or four characteristic types of social behaviour i.e. cohesive, disruptive, dependent and isolate. The psycho-dynamic or depth aspect was touched on in Chapter viii when considering how the BFA (basic family attitudes or early attitudes to the parental figures, etc.) are "introjected" into the personality as a core around which later influences are precipitated. How later they are projected in one's attitudes to people (BIA), in one's opinions and ambitions: in the leitmotif or pattern of one's life: in the things that give a sense of security, in one's manner of striving for them and in one's characteristic behaviour when deprived of them.

Below one has essayed a simple classification which considers the 3 types of social behaviour discussed in Chapter x but with the extra dimension of depth i.e. psychodynamically as well as sociodynamically. Its purposes are:—

a To classify the commoner types of reaction to the interviewer.

b To provide material for quantitative estimates in psychological profiles, ratings, etc. that may later be submitted to statistical analysis.

c To help the medical psychologist redress the balance of his experience by directing his attention to the whole range of adjustment, including the top end.

d To aid communication not only between psychologist and psychologist (whether "fixated" to a "school" or an exclusive jargon or no) but also between psychologist and the "job-analysis" and other co-workers on psychological projects.

The 3 suggested types of social personality are:—

1 the mature co-operative or objective personality (which one might abbreviate to MATCOP),

2 the immature–aggressive personality (IMAG),

3 the immature-dependent personality (IMDEP).

The Mature Co-operative or Objective Personality (MATCOP)

MATCOP is group-cohesive and derives from a BFA in which there has been a relatively happy identification with strong and kind father and mother figures. Because he has found it easy to work with—and respect—his parents in the prototypic group i.e. the family, so he finds it easy as an adult to like people and co-operate with them. His desire to maintain the family group, rather than disrupt it, grows in the adult into an urge to be group-cohesive rather than group-disruptive: to expect cohesion, to regard it as a norm and to help maintain it.

The benignity of the relationship with the parents will have made it easier to control such ambivalent (i.e. compound of simultaneous affection and resentment) reactions as have arisen in the course of parental discipline and training. It will be easier for him to avoid excessive resentment or undue dependence and to think objectively: easier to identify himself happily and spontaneously with leadership which his BFA enables him to sense as strong and understanding and therefore good. He will

F*

be better prepared to balance his willingness to co-operate with the group as follower (i.e. identified with the son-father role) with his readiness to accept a role of leadership (i.e. identified with the father-son role).

He is neither predominantly egocentric nor group-hypersensitive but is able to polarise constructively and creatively the needs of Ego and Group. In short, a cohesive BIA—deriving from a cohesive pattern of BFA—helps him to implement such potential functional level as he possesses.

MATCOP's reaction to frustration of moderate degree is in the nature of a simple—stimulating but not paralysing—anxiety until the solution has been initiated: an anxiety which makes him energetic and resourceful rather than compulsive or inhibited. An attempt to describe in further detail the signs by which he may be recognised and distinguished is made in the subsequent section on "Five Signs of a Robust Sanity". It seems important that we should be able to diagnose a high degree of sanity in our actual or potential leaders. One of the inevitable and fortunate aspects of leadership is that it must for the most part be chosen: some responsibility for leadership must rest therefore on those who choose.

The Immature aggressive Personality (IMAG)

IMAG is group-disruptive and derives from a BFA of excessive resentment and distrust: possibly of the father, of a father-mother relationship which has failed to give a sense of security, of a dominant possessive mother (not sufficiently so to induce dependency): possibly from an identification with a dominant resentfully aggressive father, etc.

The pattern of his BFA which tends to disrupt the family group—leads to a BIA whose leitmotif is to achieve a sense of security by surpassing and dominating others; by compelling an admiring submission if at all possible. His urge will be to rebel against those whose seniority or authority represent for him the resented father figure. In short, the disruptive BFA leads to a disruptive BIA.

IMAG's emotional reaction to people is one of ambivalence in which the desire for affection and interdependence is suppressed and the resentment and hatred is all too easily projected. When frustrated, he becomes more egocentric, rebellious, challenging, recalcitrant, obstinate, tactless and domineering.

While not well adapted to the group as human beings, he may—as an excuse to dominate and an opportunity to gain prestige—identify himself with what he may regard as the group purpose. He is often relatively more effective in life than IMDEP because his energies are directed outwardly into competitive activities: but it will be at the cost of an increased, incommensurate and exhausting compulsive effort and the emotional satisfaction that accrues will be relatively slight.

His desire to dominate will make him drive both himself and others: and when this compensatory drive fails, his maladjustment or neurosis takes on a self-compulsive or compulsive-obsessional colouring. With deeper frustration, his depression will be associated with much self-hate, remorse and guilt.

The Immature-dependent Personality (IMDEP)

IMDEP is group-dependent or isolate and derives from such BFA's as: emotional fixation to—and overdependence on—the mother figure, with a need for continuous reassuring love and emotional help: where both parents are themselves immature, erratic, unpredictable, neurotic or incompatible and the atmosphere and example set is one of continuous insecurity.

IMDEP'S emotional reaction to people is—as in all immature types—markedly ambivalent. But unlike IMAG, it is the aggressive component of that ambivalence that is suppressed and the appeal for affection that is too easily projected. The suppressed aggression is directed against himself with the result that when frustrated he easily lapses into depression and self-depreciation.

Ordinarily IMDEP will lean on the group or be carried by it. He attempts to please, tends to capitalise his helplessness and to cadge for help: to use charm and self-depreciating facetiousness to disarm criticism. He is over-sensitive to the group but too preoccupied about self to be consistently aware of the group-purpose. Though friendly, over-conciliatory and even submissive, he is not essentially or actively co-operative.

If his contact is poor, his compensatory abilities and drive not sufficient, the emotional help he craves not forthcoming and some sort of sociotherapeutic or psychotherapeutic help not available, he may drift from the group and become "isolate", severely inhibited or "shut-in". The "isolate" is really a variety of IMDEP.

IMDEP's reactions to frustration in the group task or interview are: shyness, simple anxiety, self-depreciation and excuse-making, defensive facetiousness, display of helplessness, etc.: if acutely demoralised he may lapse into a solipsistic isolation. His neurotic maladjustments are likely to be hysterical or anxious or psychosomatic rather than the compulsive-obsessional reactions of IMAG. With deeper frustration, his depression will be associated with a narcissistic anxiety due to fear for self, rather than by remorse and guilt as with IMAG.

C—ANALYSING—AND ALLOWING FOR—YOUR REACTION
TO THE CANDIDATE: THE COUNTER-TRANSFERENCE

The way you feel about a candidate i.e. your counter-transference is—when objectively analysed—an important source of information. Its value will depend on (a) the range of types you have experience of, (b) the degree of objectivity with which you are able to analyse that counter-transference.

It is demanded of the medical psychologist as a vocational *conditio sine qua non* that he achieve a high degree of objectivity in his judgements: which means *not* that he should be free from prejudices—which is hardly possible—but that he should know how to allow for them. It has been said that the best scientists are those who recognise their mistakes most quickly in order to correct them: it might be said that the best psychologists are those who recognise their prejudices most quickly in order to allow for them.

What the medical psychologist still lacks—especially in view of his increasingly preventive and constructive role in the community—is a sufficient experience of those whose adjustment to life is very superior. He will have much knowledge of IMDEP and IMAG types (perhaps more of the former) but such knowledge as he will have of MATCOP personalities will be on a conscious and superficial level which throws little light on their psychodynamics.

Unless he redresses the balance and extends his experience to include the top end of the scale, he will be working—as one found oneself until the obvious remedy suggested itself—with a *concept* based on unverified hypothesis and suggested by negative examples: rather than to a *clinical scale* drawn from an experience of personality over its entire range of adjustment and maturity. His criterion of "what" will be based largely on observation and experience of "what not".

Selection on leadership level with the WOSB type of procedure gives him a unique opportunity of correcting the imbalance: if he uses it wisely. If he makes a point of seeing that at least 10 per cent of his interviews are of mature and superior types, then a critical analysis of the paper screening, observation during the impasses of a leaderless group task, an interview at length, more selective observation in the group, noting and even measuring the reactions of the rest of the group, sharing the observations of other observers who are making a bearing from a different angle, all these cannot but add immeasurably to his understanding of those who adjust on the very highest levels.

In this way, he can help to build a positive concept of physical, mental and social health and happiness which may be invaluable to the community. He will explode the facile myth of leadership as a mystery in which one either is or is not invested: and will reveal it as a human function which like every other human function, though it be given by God, must be cherished by man.

In very general terms, one feels more at ease with the good candidates and less at ease with the poor ones. One may not find IMDEP, IMAG and MATCOP falling into the simplistic categories of the shy, the sullen and the spontaneous: candidates do not fall for the most part into clear-cut types as will be pointed out later in this chapter. But the good candidates will tend to be franker, friendlier, more spontaneous, more objective and co-operative, more able to contribute to an effective interview. The poor candidates will tend to be less frank and more defensive: ambivalent i.e. blowing hot and cold, either gushful or over-conciliatory or "sticky" and of high emotional viscosity: less able to disentangle their egocentric preoccupations from the demands and rights of others: less cooperative, less essentially courteous and less effective in contributing their share to the interview.

There are those one likes and respects: those one likes but does not respect: those one respects but does not like: those one neither likes nor respects. One can be definite about the first and last, fairly definite about the second: it is with the third one experiences difficulty.

D—FIVE SIGNS OF A "ROBUST SANITY"

This section is essentially an extension of section B, and especially of what has been said about MATCOP. It is an attempt to formulate a few clinical pointers which may lead to a recog-

nition of MATCOP and which may be rated in a simple way—
by a 3-point rating—so as to enable others to use, test, validate
and improve them.

Group-cohesiveness and leadership are positive functions and
in considering the sort of personality needed on leadership level,
one needs psychological help that will identify and certify something more positive than a freedom from manifest psychiatric
disability or from powerful and disturbing complexes. Until
recently the medical psychologist has had insufficient incentive,
and the general psychologist insufficient clinical experience, to
consider personality more positively. The work of the former has,
willy-nilly, been therapeutic and—too much of it—semi-custodial
rather than preventive and constructive and he has been given
little opportunity of considering personality other than in terms
of maladaptive processes.

The general psychologist has only recently begun to leave the
academic field in any number. Most of his extra-mural and
clinical experience has been in job-analysis and aptitude testing,
and more recently in the clinic and on the selection board. In
default of sufficient clinical experience of men meeting, and continuing to meet, the stresses of a living community, he has tended
to rely on the clinical experience of the medical psychologist for
his concepts of the emotional and social aspects of personality.
Neither has as yet been able to offer more positive concepts: nor
does it seem likely that they will until they combine with the
statistician, and work in team on psychological projects of the
WOSB type.

One found it difficult to meet the positive aim of selecting
potential leaders with a negative concept of personality and with
an experience of human adjustment somewhat heavily loaded on
the lower levels of effectiveness. Fortunately the nature of the
material provided an unique opportunity of redressing the
balance of one's experience. One was dealing in the first instance
with potential officers pre-selected mainly from the top 10 per
cent of the population so far as measurable general intelligence
was concerned. All were screened intensively from the written
material and tests and observed in Stress Group Tasks. One
made a point of devoting from 10 per cent upwards of one's interviews to the very cream of the candidature, the best in each batch,
any that seemed outstanding; those of extremely high potential
level as indicated by an OIR of 10 or 9 (roughly corresponding

in the intelligence scale to the top in 800 and in 260 respectively in the general population). One had the additional opportunity, for over a year, of assisting in the selection of commissioned officers of successful experience and superior ability for special jobs in Parachute and Glider Regiments, as Personnel Selection Officers for WOSB and for other purposes.

It was not possible to observe so many superior candidates so intensively for so long without noting a great deal of spontaneous and characteristic social behaviour. Nor could one help acquiring a clinical sense or "feel" of the differences between well-adjusted and poorly-adjusted group members. One did not resist the temptation to differentiate this clinical "feel" into its components and to formulate them in positive terms.

Statistical procedure cannot formulate hypotheses, it can merely test them. Hypotheses about personality traits and roles can derive usefully only from clinical observation of men behaving and reacting in the living context of the group. If such hypothetical traits are quantitatively estimated—even in a 3-point rating—there should be no difficulty in testing their practical usefulness and their validity: and they may serve as springboard to a more precisely differentiated concept of personality. Such provisional hypotheses as the nature of one's work suggested seemed to serve one usefully, to relate helpfully to one's clinical judgements and conclusions, and to provide a practical and simple means of helping others to acquire skill in judgement.

One will suggest therefore as signs of the mature or socially superior personality—signs one might say of a "robust sanity" or of MATCOP—the following

1 WARMTH of Feeling,
2 SPONTANEITY of Expressive Behaviour,
3 OBJECTIVITY of Social Thinking,
4 CO-OPERATIVENESS of Social Behaviour,
5 COMMENSURATE EFFECTIVENESS of Total—including Functional—Behaviour.

The first two can be sensed even in the early phases of the interview: the third may usually be elicited after some discussion: the fourth and fifth may be estimated from the paper screening and interview in combination with the observation of test behaviour.

Each sign will be considered in terms of a 3-point rating of

Plus (+), Zero (0) and Minus (−): which could easily become a
5-point rating by adding a Double Plus and a Double Minus.
From a 3-point rating of all 5 signs one has sufficient material
for a 3-point global rating of Social Maturity which will be discussed at the end of this section. Social Maturity—as here considered—is a slightly wider concept than group-cohesiveness, for
it also considers the commensurateness of group-effectiveness.

Under the Plus rating will be considered the actual positive
sign: under the Minus rating, its polar opposite, or perhaps more
correctly its "scalar" extreme: under the Zero rating will be
considered just a sufficient degree of the positive sign to enable
the individual to function adequately and cope reasonably.

Each sign is considered as distributed in a graduated series
of which both ends constitute scalar extremes: there is therefore
no dichotomy of the mature and the immature. Moreover the
mature or superior personality is *not* in the middle: is *not* clustered
round the mean or average in the series: he is at the top end
of the scale. It is for this reason that one dislikes the bipolar
scales which place virtue—in respect of any quality—intermediately between two polar vices or extremes. Virtue lies in the
most effective adaptation—not in the most intermediate. The
Aristotelian Golden Mean is a venerable tightrope conception
which seems to deny two negatives, two scalar extremes, rather
than to affirm a useful positive: and may have led to muddled
thinking. While personality may be the result of a polarisation
and wedding of opposing dynamic trends, it cannot very well be
their average.

Each sign will also be considered (a) as revealed and projected
in selection procedure (b) as exemplified in literature and in the
community generally.

WARMTH of Feeling

Perhaps the most valuable single clinical impression of the
superior candidate—the really well-adjusted individual—is of
a "warm spontaneity". The man who feels warmly and kindly
towards his fellow men does not have to compel himself to seem
friendly: his expressive muscles reveal it spontaneously without a
compulsive *moue* or conscious facial gesture. "Warmth" and
"spontaneity" very naturally go together: we will however for
the moment isolate them and consider "warmth" first.

The Plus candidate strikes one as easy, friendly, frank and
empathic: as having a greater capacity for genuine out-going

free-flowing emotional warmth. The Minus candidate strikes one as blowing alternately hot and cold, as emotionally ambivalent, as "spotty", erratic and capricious in his attitude to others. He tends to alternate between violent likes and dislikes: between defensive gush or over-conciliatory gestures and an oral-aggressive over-vehemence, irritability, obstinacy and resentment: between enthusiasms and antipathies, self-display and self-depreciation. His charm is somewhat synthetic, his conciliatoriness not without an *arrière-pensée* of veiled aggression. His empathy is defective and its selectiveness out of gear in that he is over-sensitive about his own opinions and what others think of him and under-sensitive about the feelings and emotional needs of others. Whether he manifest himself as an obvious "disruptive" or "dependent" or as overtly ambivalent will depend on the relative strengths of the conflicting needs for dominance and dependence.

In the last issue, the only true dynamic of spontaneous and natural social effort is this natural out-going warmth of MATCOP which ordinarily derives from a good cohesive BFA but which may be otherwise achieved with effort, sacrifice and help. To the extent that a man cannot like people or trust them or want to work with them, to that extent he cannot co-operate spontaneously and his social effort becomes a compulsive drive rather than a zestful urge and outflowing. He cannot be kind: the moment compulsion relaxes, aggression and resentment step forward. His gush and his charm and his conciliatory attitudes are compulsive and calculated attempts to conceal or antidote his resentment. He may achieve at great cost a high degree of conscientious consideration for others, a compulsive benignity: but its stability will be slight, its objectivity small and—lacking the single-hearted warmth of true kindness—it will slump too readily into severity. His is the ambivalence which derives from the BFA of the child which has been excessively dependent on its parents or dominated by them and which has resented being dependent or dominated.

Considering "warmth" in terms of a 3-point rating, one may describe the Plus candidate as a "warm personality", the Zero candidate as "on the whole friendly and approachable" and the Minus candidate as "predominantly ambivalent" i.e. erratic and unpredictable, "difficult", critical, intolerant, prickly, angular, cold or even "shut-in".

As pointers to the presence or absence of this warmth, we have already discussed the interpretation of the Projective Battery. The Human Problems Session will give a clear indication: so will the Judgement Test, though one will have to make some allowance for the "group equation" (page 206). The best indicator of all is the analysis of one's own counter-transference: a warm counter-transference in the interviewer is likely to be part of one's response to a warm transference and frank friendly manner in the interviewee.

Perhaps the best, most convincing exemplar of the warm personality in literature is Alyosha in Dostoevsky's "Brothers Karamazov". Alyosha's is a capacity for warm rich affection and compassion which wells up spontaneously from a warm heart: there is in it no trace of the compulsions of guilt or the urges of a spiritual narcissism: it is not the erethistic, hyperfastidious over sensitiveness of a compulsive benignity which is concerned in reality more with the doer of good than with the target of his goodness. (We will not however attempt to relate it to his BFA).

Alyosha has all the calm of true compassion which transmutes all its empathic suffering into constructive help, and fritters none of it away in spiritual and emotional malaise. His is a real compassion, not a compensatory and guilty oversensitiveness: it manifests itself naturally, sweetly and without impediment: its "spontaneity" is the second sign of mental and social and spiritual health which we will go on to discuss.

Spontaneity of Expressive Behaviour

We have called attention to the co-existence of "warmth" and "spontaneity" as one's most valuable single clinical impression of the superior candidate. And have suggested that psychodynamically this is because a man who likes people and feels an emotional need to participate in their social efforts will do so spontaneously: whereas, if he feels ambivalently and has no single-hearted desire to co-operate, he will have to compel himself to do so.

How does this spontaneity manifest itself?

Ordinarily emotions and emotional attitudes manifest themselves in the so-called expressive muscular movements. Of these, facial expression, speech and gesture are the basic triad. But some expressive function is served in muscular function generally: in posture, movement, dancing, handwriting, etc.

A warm friendly attitude—free from any strong streak of

ambivalence—will, for example, tend to manifest itself in facial expression that is mobile and relaxed: in gestures that are fluid, expansive and outward rather than rigid, constricted and inward: in a voice of flexible and lively range: in speech that is without hesitation: in a calligraphy that is free-flowing and forward-moving rather than cramped, tense and slow to advance: in movements that are easy, natural and unforced: and generally in an easy balance of posture and movement.

A strongly ambivalent attitude to people will determine a different muscular and expressive pattern. Facial expression will be fixed either in a compulsive semblance or *moue* of determination or goodwill or, in an inhibited poker face. Speech will be monotonously lacking in range of pitch, volume, tempo or emphasis though it may be overvehement on a single note. There may be a forced "press" of speech or it may be hesitant: stammering is often associated with the repression of strong aggressive impulses. The calligraphy will show some element of compulsive tension: it may be cramped, angular, erratic in direction or slope: it may alternately press forward or lag behind: a word or line will begin with a forward slope and end with a backward one. Movement and posture will be tense, rigid and awkward: sometimes to the extent of constituting accident-proneness.

What is the scalar extreme to spontaneity?

To the schematist it might seem to be inhibition: but clinically —as the manifestations described above suggest—it would seem to be a behavioral complex of compulsive and inhibitory elements. Psychiatric usage commonly restricts the word "compulsive" to a "press" of activity: it might equally well be applied to a forced inhibition of activity: there may be a compulsion to do— or *not* to do.

Certainly in the "compulsive-obsessional" reaction and personality, this association of compulsive press or drive with compulsive inhibition seems to exist. It seems to correspond psychodynamically to the phasic predominance of aggressive or submissive elements in the ambivalent attitude to people. If aggressiveness prevails, it will find vent in behaviour with a compulsive tinge: if it is suppressed, the ability to exteriorise emotion in expressive movements may be inhibited with it.

In a Hamlet, for instance, the compulsion *not* to do is powerful and in the play almost prevails: in a Lady Macbeth the compulsion to do cannot be resisted. Both react ambivalently and compulsively and without spontaneity.

At one end of this scale is the spontaneous natural urge to co-operate with one's fellow men: at the other end is the forced drive of the ambivalent which results in compulsive pressures and compulsive inhibitions. At this ambivalent end, the balance between these conflicting pressures and inhibitions is necessarily unstable: there will be indecisive phases where there may be intermediate anxious strivings to convert an inhibition into a compulsion or *vice versa:* and these indecisive phases may be characterised by the "teetering" anxiety which can never be far from the mind of the ambivalent.

When spontaneity dies, compulsion takes over: with the death of desire, craving takes command. The spontaneity and zest and appetite of the natural urge give way to the compulsions, inhibitions, zestlessness and insatiable neurotic craving of the forced drive.

From the easy spontaneity of the well-adjusted, three forms of behaviour must be distinguished:—

a The uninhibited babbling of the immature or naïf: in whom there may be a slight compulsive press due to the burgeoning of instincts over which additional control has not yet been acquired. They are not so much at their ease as over-excited and slightly confused.

b The overactive elation of the pathologically uninhibited hypomanic cycloids or "mood-swingers" who are the "life and death of any party". They should be recognised at any selection board and promptly referred to the medical psychologist. They produce an uneasy counter-transference and to the trained clinician there is a strong "smell" of smouldering aggression.

c The blarney of the synthetic charmer which is more rehearsed and acted than spontaneous: and not at all warm.

In a 3-point rating, the Plus candidate may be described as "spontaneous", the Zero candidate as "fairly natural in manner," the Minus candidate as "inhibited and/or compulsive, possibly indecisive".

The Human Problems Session and Undirected Group Discussion will quickly reveal spontaneity in speech. Important screening clues will come from the Projection Battery, especially the WAT. Most valuable of all will be the interview, where the degree of spontaneity reached—and the cost in effort to the interviewer—provides an excellent index.

An interesting related concept is the Zen concept of "Muga" associated with the principle of "Wu-wei" (page 157).

Muga ("no self" or "absence of self") is the absence of the feeling "I am doing it". In Judo wrestling, in fencing, in painting, in the Japanese Tea Ceremony it expresses itself in a non-interfering attitude which allows not a hairsbreadth between thought and action. The analogy is used of the hands when clapped: the sound which issues does so without deliberation, without hesitation, without interruption for conscious thought: there is no mediacy: in Muga, speed is never aimed at but is always the result of the immediacy of the reaction.

The Muga concept passed over—via the Sung painting of Hangchow—to the Kano school of Japan: finding in the Sumiye (black and white) genre its highest expression.

Sumiye is painting with black chinese ink and a soft yielding brush on thin fragile paper or silk. With these materials, the artist is compelled to draw quickly, without hesitation, blot or erasure; without repetition, correction or re-touching: once executed, the strokes are indelible and irrevocable. If the artist's spontaneity ceases, an ugly blot appears, the paper is torn and his work is spoiled. It is this spontaneity and flowing immediacy that catches things alive and gives the work freshness and living movement: yet it also compels an underlying calm and poise so as to eliminate non-essentials; and the utmost sharpening and awareness of all one's faculties. The principle of Muga was applied to the practical arts of painting, Judo wrestling, fencing and the Tea Ceremony: but, according to the Zenist, life itself should be lived as spontaneously—and as calmly, fastidiously, and intensely—as the Sumiye artist paints his picture.

It is to be noted that the spontaneity of Muga and Zen is no mere withdrawal or lack of inhibition: it is the natural unforced expression of the balanced and disciplined and overflowing personality: it results from a creative polarisation of immediacy and spontaneity on the one hand with mastery and a sharpened awareness and control on the other. Such a balance—such an "at-oneness" with one's experience—may occur on any level from Shakespeare down to the simplest individual who is socially mature on his own level: perhaps this spontaneity is the spark of creativeness that exists in every man.

In literary art, Shakespeare is perhaps the outstanding exemplar of that polarisation of spontaneity and mastery at the highest level of human imaginative expression. Though his imaginative power was supreme, there seems to be no internal or external evidence to suggest that he laboured unduly.

In the art of living generally, Goethe is surely the richest exemplar. In poetry, love, human affairs and government, science, philosophy and art—indeed in every aspect of a rich life and in every phase of a long and fruitful one until his death at 82— he combined freshness and intensity of experience with profundity and completeness of understanding. Though Shakespeare was the greater poet, Goethe was the greater man.

Objectivity of Social Thinking

Objectivity—the third sign—may be defined in its most general terms as the ability to distinguish and relate the interests of Self and Group in one's thinking. Its scalar extreme will be egocentric, self-centred or emotional thinking.

To expand this definition slightly, a first requirement of the objective attitude is the ability to dissociate, balance, reconcile and ultimately bind the interests and needs of the Self and the Group into a fruitful relationship to meet a common challenge, group-purpose or LOTS.

A second requirement is the ability to make the necessary allowance for the emotional and personal bias in one's thinking. Emotion may be directed to animate one's activities but should not be allowed to confuse one's thinking. It is not a question of trying to eliminate the personal reaction but of acquiring insight into its nature and degree so that one may allow for it. One should for instance—to take a very relevant and practical issue in leadership—be able to dissociate one's liking or dislike for a man from one's estimate of his functional ability to serve the group-purpose: an ability which the Judgement Test sets out to evaluate.

In committee, emotional egocentric thinking makes a man fixated to his early preconceptions or first opinions because he fears that a semblance of inconsistency may subtract from his prestige. The objective thinker identifies himself with the changing problem and not primarily with the impression his opinion creates. One noticed in WOSB conferences that the objective team-member, once he saw the relevance or justness of an opinion different to his own, changed his mind almost before the sentence was finished.

Commonsense is surely objectivity in the sense used here: if the word does really mean something and is not merely a semantic trick to suggest that my doxy—being commonsense—automatically becomes orthodoxy while your doxy must needs be heterodoxy. Emotional thinking may so depreciate the judgement of a superior intellect that it is in effect no better than that of an inferior intelligence. That is, of course, no argument in favour of the inferior intelligence: the objective commonsense of an OIR 10 must be considerably superior to the commonsense of the OIR 1 or "average" man. It is the emotional interference—not the intelligence—that is at fault.

Objectivity and Humour

An important indicator of a man's objectivity, of his sense of perspective in human relationships, is the way in which he—consciously or unconsciously—uses humour: whether to defend himself, attack others or de-tense the situation.

Oral-aggressive humour is generally an attempt to disrupt and demoralise an individual or group: that at any rate will be its ultimate effect. Defensive, self-depreciative humour may in its milder form be an attempt to de-tense oneself momentarily in order to regain one's poise. It may be—and often is—an attempt to disarm criticism and evade responsibility.

The mature objective use of humour is to de-tense a situation where there is conflict between the demands of the group and the needs of the individual. In moments of stress it aims to de-tense the group or an individual or oneself. Its effect will be to reduce interpersonal friction in the group and intrapsychic friction in the individual.

Both aggressive and defensive humour are relatively immature. The maturest most objective use of humour is of good intent and aims to raise the morale, functional efficiency and ultimate well-being of men and groups.

The most specific method of actually testing a candidate's objectivity in judging others is provided by the Judgement Test. The estimate of his own performance elicited in this test when combined with the "Self-description" of the Projection Battery will give useful pointers to his objectivity in judging himself. The Human Problems Session and the interview will however make the major contribution to an estimate of objectivity.

In a 3-point rating, the Plus candidate "has good objectivity" and is capable of a realistic evaluation of people and jobs and himself. The Zero candidate "has moderate objectivity": or, if immature because of age or inexperience, has developed as well as may reasonably be expected in the right direction (unlike "warmth" and "spontaneity", objectivity can only reach full development with full adulthood). The Minus candidate "is capable of little objectivity and is not able to allow for the emotional elements in his thinking". He may be a "blimp" (predisposed to project his aggression and to blame others long before himself), a "self-blamer" (predisposed to blame, depreciate or underestimate himself), prejudiced, intolerant, erratic and influenced by mood, suggestible and over-influenced by the opinions of others, etc., etc.

An unusually fine literary examplar of objectivity on its very highest level is the Guru in the remarkable novel by L. H. Myers in two volumes i.e. *The Root and the Flower* and *The Pool of Vishnu*. This is of such rare insight and wisdom and valid on so many levels—quite apart from the distinction of its writing—that no advanced psychotherapist could fail to be stimulated by it: especially by " The Story of Mohan and Damayanti" in the second volume, in itself a case-history rich in the wisdom of therapy. The Indian background is merely a technical device to create a timeless setting free from topical associations, against which the recurrent patterns of human relationships and emotions can be projected.

The role of the Guru corresponds, in Western terms, largely to that of the psychotherapist; of whom the nature of his work demands the highest degree of objectivity: and that he be, not perfect, but aware of his imperfections. In the story, he is represented as no smug paragon of immaculate infallibility but as a very human, very fallible, very wise old man who—because of a rare combination of intelligence, knowledge, experience and compassion derived from his own past and present suffering—wishes to share his wisdom with all who may benefit from it: with no pretence to moral superiority but in all humility.

A distinguished scientist has said that he makes just as many mistakes as his pupils but corrects more of them. Similarly, the more objective individual is not necessarily freer from emotional thinking: but is able—and accustomed—to allow for those emotional elements that tend to distort his judgements. The objectivity of the Guru is of this type: his true superiority in spiritual stature is no static one, born of eliminated and out-lived desires, but an ever-striving one which grows as much by its failures as by its victories.

CO-OPERATIVENESS of Social Behaviour

Co-operativeness—the fourth sign—is the urge and desire to bind one's own interests with that of the group: to earn the group's approval and enjoy its friendship by making positive contributions to its purposes and aims. It will derive very naturally from a warm BIA; and its implementation constitutes much of the group-cohesiveness with which WOSB so largely concerns itself.

At the other scalar extreme is uncooperativeness which may manifest itself in an antisocial desire to dominate or disrupt the group: or failing that, to depend parasitically on it: or in the last resort—if the attempt to maintain contact proves too difficult—to cut completely away from it. In short we have again the disruptive, the dependent and the isolate.

The Plus candidate is objective enough to balance the interests of Self and Group and to give proper weight to each. He is therefore relatively less ego-centred and more group-centred. The Minus candidate, because of his ambivalence, is inclined to see life—not as a co-operative activity—but as a battle in which one takes the attack and tries to dominate: if one cannot do that, one is a passive resister or a passive dependent: in the last resort one may have to retire from a lost battle.

In a 3-point rating, the Plus candidate is "actively co-operative", the Zero candidate is "helpful and willing to join in" the Minus candidate is "disruptive, dependent or isolate."

The leaderless group tasks are specially designed to project the candidate's cooperativeness as implemented in his group-cohesiveness. The biography will provide clues in the number of social clubs, societies, sports teams, etc. he has joined and the offices he has held.

One of the better results of the good boarding-school—so

WOSB experience clearly shows—is the opportunity it gives to learn to respect and enjoy the larger group from an early stage in one's social and emotional development. No doubt an ideal home which took an active part in the community life around it would be better still. But at the age when they are seen at WOSB (18 to 19), the boarding-school candidate is generally more mature socially than the day-school boy. What happens after that has not, so far as one knows, been investigated.

"Team-mindedness"—as distinct from a heightened suggestibility to higher authority which makes for regimentation—is traditionally a British characteristic. This urge to balance the individual and his personality with the group within which he functions freely—an urge not yet used to its full—is an important part of Britain's contribution to civilisation. It is not a compromise between the individual and the team: it is a creative polarisation of both.

COMMENSURATE EFFECTIVENESS of Total—including Functional-Behaviour

Commensurate effectiveness—the fifth sign—is an effect of the preceding four. It is the ratio between the candidate's total actual efficiency (both functional and social) and his potential efficiency.

The Plus candidate is one who contributes effectively and spontaneously on his own commensurate level and in his own field. He may be rated as "effective".

The contribution of the Zero ("adequate") candidate will be:—

a adequate but not reasonably commensurate with his potential ability;
b if commensurate, achieved with disproportionate effort and therefore with a diminishment of stability;
c commensurate occasionally but not consistently;
d commensurate in some sub-fields but not in others.

The contribution of the Minus ("ineffective") candidate will be:—

a never better than adequate but inconsistently so, even with increased effort;
b adequate with such disproportionate effort as to impair his stability and reliability seriously;
c completely ineffective on the level to be expected.

Commensurate effectiveness (CE) is of course not the same as Group-effectiveness (GE). The latter is a measure of his absolute level i.e. whether on or below officer level: the former is the ratio between his actual GE and his potential GE and is the measure therefore of his success in adjustment, of his social maturity. It will be estimated from his past record and present showing.

A MATCOP whose CE is high but whose GE is low may be quite unable to function on leadership level. An IMDEP or IMAG may, despite a personality handicap, have a sufficiently high GE to so function without serious strain or instability: though his GE will of course be correspondingly diminished.

The classic literary example of extreme "commensurate ineffectiveness" is "Oblomov" in the novel by Goncharov which gives the name of "Oblomovism" to the futility of the man who has developed his intellect and sensitivity at the cost of every other active and social human quality: and who remains therefore an emotionally infantile personality.

The "highbrow" has been defined as one "educated above his intelligence": of Oblomov one might say that he has been educated well above and beyond his character and emotional maturity. He talks eternally of plans, projects, ideas and ambitions but does nothing to implement them. When the failing sympathy and established boredom of even his best friends cease to supply him with the vicarious and temporary sense of power that he derives from being listened to, he takes to his bed: there to dream without impediment—day in, day out—grander and nobler dreams which no reality will ever be required to test. He is half way towards that private phantasy world which is schizophrenia.

Five Pairs of Antinomies

These signs with their extremes resolve themselves into five pairs of antinomies. Between each sign and its antinomy, people may be evaluated in terms of a series—possibly of Gaussian distribution—but certainly not in terms of an absolute dichotomy or trichotomy. The use of a 3-point rating for each pair merely superimposes a formal trichotomy—supplying convenient points of reference—on what is essentially a series. These five pairs are not intended to represent exclusive categories or comprise a complete classification of dynamic personality traits: they are intended merely to represent the facets of characteristic social behaviour and feeling most likely to strike the observer. They may be listed as follows:—

1 *Warmth of feeling* . . . . *ambivalence.*
2 *Spontaneity* of expressive behaviour i.e. of speech, facial expression, gesture, writing, movement and posture, etc. . . . . *compulsiveness*, manifest either positively as a compulsive press or negatively as a compulsive inhibition.
3 *Objectivity* of social thinking i.e. the ability to distinguish and relate the interests of Self and Group . . . . *egocentric* self-centred *or emotional thinking.*
4 *Co-operativeness* of social behaviour . . . . the *uncooperativeness* of the disruptive, dependent or isolate.
5 *Commensurate effectiveness* of total—including functional— behaviour i.e. actual group-effectiveness as compared with potential group-effectiveness . . . . *ineffectiveness.*

E—A 3-POINT RATING OF SOCIAL MATURITY

A 3-point global rating of social maturity, based on the above five signs with any other relevant information, can usefully crystallise one's clinical impressions in a form usable in psychological ratings and profiles and for the evaluation of stability (page 181).

The Plus candidate, in terms of this global rating is reasonably warm, spontaneous, objective, co-operative and effective in relation to his ability and the effort he makes. These are in effect the signs of MATCOP.

The Minus candidate is ambivalent and uncertain in mood: may drive himself compulsively or suffer from crippling inhibitions of activity: thinks too much in terms of self and lets this influence his planning: is a poor co-operator because of a predisposition to be either dominating and disruptive or dependent: his effectiveness is seriously diminished by the strains of overcompensating effort, poor social contact, etc. These are in effect signs of IMAG or IMDEP.

Striking laterally across this vertical scale of adjustment and at its lower end, these unbalanced immature ambivalent personalities, IMAG and IMDEP, constitute a lateral series of their own. At one end of this lateral series, the aggressive component of ambivalence is predominantly directed outwards in IMAG:

at the other end, it is predominantly directed inwards in IMDEP. The position in the series will depend on the extent to which one or other of these components (aggressiveness or submissiveness) predominates.

In practice, a 3-point rating of this kind is both simple and useful. While the greater number of candidates may not crystallise into patterns so clearly marked as those schematised above, there will be no difficulty in deciding those whose pattern is definitely good and definitely bad. The Zero candidate will have a sufficient degree of the positive signs to assist—on the whole—in the implementation of his potential ability.

The Signs of Superior and Poor Groups

After observing a large number of experimental groups intensively for short periods and a small number of observer teams for much longer periods, one noted that superior and poor groups or teams have characteristics not unlike those of superior and poor group members: at any rate there are certain analogies. And one can often sense the atmosphere and quality of a group within 5 minutes of meeting it.

The "blimpish" IMAG type of team quickly reveals in its conversation a tendency to the oral-aggressive use of humour which manifests itself in argument, debate, teasing, chaffing and bickering: in attempts—in the guise of play—to make others lose face while elevating one's own individual prestige in the group: in humour used combatively and destructively and *not* as a means of de-tensing the group and its individual members in order to encourage and induce a constructive solution of its problems and enquiries on a higher level of effectiveness. Characteristic of it is the way in which it "blimps" or projects the aggression due to its own frustration and incapacity on others, on other —possibly weaker—members of the team or on those it judges. It is apt to be intolerant, uncharitable and psychologically obtuse, especially with those it has difficulty in understanding.

Because of this ambivalence of attitude, the poor or socially immature team is not really spontaneous. Its compulsiveness reveals itself in an uneasy over-vehemence and dogmatism and in an inhibition of the free and spontaneous play of opinion, especially in members who are younger or weaker or junior (by rank). There is a tendency—especially in older or senior members, but it soon infects the younger—to identify oneself too fixedly with opinions once expressed rather than to relate them flexibly to the clarifying situation: in short, to equate consistency with one's first impression with consistency of character and force of intellect.

The IMAG atmosphere conduces to strong likes and dislikes, erratic and uncharitable judgements and little objectivity: to disintegration into sub-groups or cliques; aiming to outvote each other rather than at a co-operative pooling of resources and a decision by general agreement. It produces—in the young and the emotionally retarded—the individual who, in a petty way, is "power-drunk" with the authority vested in him to influence or decide the fate of others: rather than humbled by its responsibility. Such a team shows a relative inability to co-ordinate its collective intelligence, experience and energy into constructive effective action. One or two strong members of an otherwise poor group may infect it with maturity and alter its quality: that is of course where the highest leadership lies.

The really superior MATCOP group has a warm tolerant zestful atmosphere which encourages completely spontaneous speech, behaviour and improvisation of ideas in all of its members. Argument, with its killing of constructive thought and cooperative effort, its unproductive and time-consuming sparring for prestige, gives way to a more creative discussion: prejudices and biases are freely admitted, vented and allowed for. The individual member is allowed and expected to change his opinions freely and keep his judgement fluid until he has considered all the evidence and all the opinions. No prestige is attached to a rigid identification with one's first impressions: much is attached to one's ability to identify oneself objectively with the changing flux of evidence. The MATCOP team is on the whole likelier to co-ordinate and relate its collective capacity, experience and energy to the effective solution of its problems.

The collective intelligence of a crowd or mob is notoriously poorer than that of many of the individuals in it, though the strength of its collective convictions may be greater: the crowd might be said to have the courage of a lion but the intelligence of a louse. The capacity of the mature individual is greater than that of a crowd and probably greater than that of many poor groups: but it is far less than the collective capacity of a small happily co-ordinated group of mature co-operative members. A mature team liberates and amplifies as well as binds its members:

but they are more aware of its liberating and amplifying effect than of its binding effect which is accepted as an insurance of security within the effective and friendly group.

One might describe the group, as well as its members, in terms of the 5 signs of social maturity here suggested. The poor group is ambivalent in its interpersonal reactions, inhibited about some of its activities and compulsively straining about others; prone to disproportionately strong likes and dislikes and weak in objectivity; temperamentally competitive rather than co-operative; predisposed to overemphasise the vested authority that derives from a function and to underemphasise its vested responsibility: and on the whole ineffective in the use of its collective capacities. The good group is warm, spontaneous, objective, co-operative and effective in the use of its collective abilities and energies.

III—Evaluating the Candidate's Stability

If we consider stability in terms of the man, the job and the group, the questions we may ask are:—

Is his Level adequate?
Is his Group-cohesiveness adequate?
Is his Morale adequate?
Is his physical and mental Drive adequate?

The first two have already been considered: the last two have been mentioned (p. 95) and may now be considered more fully.

MORALE IN RELATION TO STABILITY

A man's effectiveness and stability at any moment are determined not only by his level, group-cohesiveness and present health but by an additional conditioning factor resulting from past experiences, achievements, failures, successes and general history. A vicious circle of consistent failure, frustration and isolation will predispose him to a continuation of failure: a virtuous circle of progressive successful achievement will predispose him to continuing success, confidence and courage.

What is Morale?

One may consider morale provisionally as a man's predisposition to success or failure, effectiveness or ineffectiveness, to do well or poorly on the level on which he should ordinarily be quite adequate; and in tasks which come within his range. It is the extent to which he is failure-prone or success-prone, lucky or unlucky.

That predisposition is the resultant of all the stabilising and unstabilising factors that have operated in his past: it is his personal Karma, his past actions and their consequences, his history determining his present. A better analogy than the circle might be the spiral: the upward clockwise virtuous spiral leading to integration of the personality, the downward anti-clockwise vicious spiral leading to disintegration and demoralisation of the personality.

Once the movement in either direction has gathered momentum—and here we will change our analogies once more —it is like the rotating flywheel whose predisposition is to continue in the direction of that momentum. The slightest push in that direction will accelerate it manifestly whereas even a strong pull will not reverse it. In this flywheel analogy, we are equating "momentum" with "predisposition" or "morale".

Morale versus Predisposition

One prefers the word "morale" to "predisposition" (much used in medico-psychological studies) for several reasons that seem important.

The first and most important is that "predisposition" has progressively acquired a loose connotation which links it too exclusively with hereditary factors: "morale" has acquired no such connotation. What many clinical studies of "predisposition" in psychiatric illnesses seem to prove—if they prove anything—is that a man whose mental health is poor (either because he is beginning to break down or has not completely recovered from a breakdown) is more likely to break down than one whose mental health is good. This very natural "predisposition"—once validated—is quoted as proof that hereditary factors are involved: which seems to be a misleading *non sequitur*.

Unloading the major part of "predisposition"—or all of it— on heredity is the relic of an older attitude in medicine, in support of which there seems to be no real evidence. It is however ceasing to be fashionable to "pass the buck" to heredity: a more fruitful concept, closer to such evidence as is available, regards hereditary and acquired factors as interacting at every phase of development; so that the resultant "predisposition" is the accumulated product of both.

A second reason is allied to the first. "Predisposition" has acquired a connotation of the static and unalterable (presumably because of its strong association with hereditary factors). That "morale" may be high or low implies that it is a changing relative dynamic process: one can envisage it being changed by the level imposed on a man by his own deliberate choice, by a selection procedure of some kind or by chance.

A third reason is that just as there is a predisposition to maladjustment, so there is a predisposition to successful adjustment. The word "predisposition" is unfortunately tainted with the former connotation: "morale" may connote either or any intermediate stage. It lends itself also to the useful concepts of neurosis as a severe demoralisation, psychosis as a complete and utter demoralisation, therapy and rehabilitation as techniques essentially for the raising of individual morale.

A fourth and important reason is that "morale" may be of the group as well as of the individual: whereas one does not easily think in terms of a group's "predisposition". It does seem reasonable to suppose a relationship between the morale of a group and that of its individual members: the former is likely to be a product of the latter. In experimental groups one notes that certain groups seem to be strongly accident-prone, while others take every risk but can apparently do no wrong.

In brief, one prefers "morale" to "predisposition" because it may be related to the group or the individual, to successful as well as to unsuccessful adjustment, to health or breakdown. It can connote both the hereditary and environmental factors that influence adjustment: and by giving a completer, more dynamic, truer picture—and one which is more in accordance with the evidence—it leads to a less fatalist attitude to instability and low morale.

Drive in Relation to Stability

After considering level, group-cohesiveness and morale in relation to effectiveness and stability, there are still a number of residual factors which the medical psychologist is aware of— and is able to make clinical judgements about—but cannot readily classify. One might tentatively group these under "drive": which we will define as "the volume and availability of energy".

There do seem to be factors which influence and determine the total volume of available energy and the tempo of using it up. Some men seem to expend their energy in large packets or "quanta" though the total volume may not be large, may even be relatively diminished: others use their energy in smaller quanta at a slower tempo but may be able to achieve an equal or greater volume of work over a longer period. The factors that determine tempo will probably also determine the rate at which a man can accelerate it and mobilise his total energies from scratch.

What seems of practical importance is that a man who is being compelled to work above his optimum tempo or beyond the volume of energy he can safely spare may be rendered thereby unstable and ultimately useless.

Such factors may be hereditary or acquired, physiological or psychological. Endocrine make-up may be largely constitutional and inherited: physical fitness and robust health is largely acquired. There are many physiological components of drive still to be fully investigated and co-ordinated. Useful further information could probably be obtained from the fuller relating of such physiological data as: the Basal Metabolic Rate, Vital Capacity and Exercise Tolerance tests: tests of endocrine, liver, kidney function: tests of muscular co-ordination, stamina and tone, etc.

Medical psychologists are well aware of the effects of anxiety and depression on the physiological reactions of heart, lungs, alimentary system, muscle etc. Its increasing recognition in general medicine is reflected in the ever-increasing field of "psychosomatic medicine": an unwise artifact, because it dissociates emotional states with a predominance of physiological concomitants from those where these concomitants are less in evidence.

Fatigue as a depression equivalent has been a clinical commonplace for years. Minor degrees of drivelessness due to minor transient or recurrent anxieties and depressions are common in the community: clinical experience and recent researches amply confirm this and suggest that their accumulative effect—in industry, for example—is considerable. These fatigue states are an indication of low morale and instability: and untreated they are a cause of further psychic infection.

There is need of further research in this field where the physiological and psychological determinants of drive interact. Exclusively physiological research has up to the moment been disappointing: medico-psychological investigation has been more fruitful: the synergistic efforts of physiologists, psychologists and statisticians—in team—should add considerably to our ability to understand, diagnose, prevent and treat states of acquired drivelessness and low morale.

Though the components of drive are not yet clearly differentiated, it is possible to make a clinical estimate of it: and the experienced medical psychologist, who is regularly required to make such estimates, is in the best position to do so.

Use of a Short Profile in Evaluating Stability

A short profile of 3-point ratings on the stability factors here discussed could be of value, (a) in helping the medical psychologist to achieve greater precision in judgement, (b) in making possible a follow-up to compare and relate these judgements with the subsequent effectiveness of the candidate.

Morale and Drive are, for the moment, probably better rated as one combined item; in which case the profile will have the following items:

1 Level: plus (+), zero (o), or minus (−).
2 Group-cohesiveness: ,, ,, ,, ,, ,, ,,
3 Morale (including
    Drive): ,, ,, ,, ,, ,, ,,
4 Global Rating of
    Stability: ,, ,, ,, ,, ,, ,,

As tentative criteria for these ratings, one suggests the following:—

1 *Level.* Candidates with OIR 6 or 7 and an Educational Standard of 3 (School Certificate Standard) are given a zero rating. Those whose OIR or ES, or both, are higher are given a plus rating. Those whose OIR or ES, or both, are below are given a minus rating. Where either is above and the other below, the candidate is given a zero rating.

2 *Group-cohesiveness.* The 3-point rating of social maturity given in this chapter may be used.

3 *Morale* (including drive).

A plus rating may be given where a man's achievements have been good in relation to his level and opportunity: especially if he displays in reasonable degree the five signs of "robust sanity" and superior adjustment given here.

A minus rating may be given:—

a if the sample of morale obtained in the "impasse" of the BS or in the interview in response to a "jolt" or stressful "silent pause" is low.

b if there is a history of anxiety, depression or "psycho-somatic" symptoms, especially when these recur at times of increased emotional stress. Such symptoms as: fatigue (unrelated to effort or disease), hay-fever, asthma, migraine, nervous dyspepsia, cardiac neurosis, stammer, enuresis, bladder frequency, hyperthyroid disorder, some cases of myositis, non-infective skin complaints, etc.

c if there is a history of actual psychiatric illness or breakdown.

4 *Global rating of Stability.* This will be based on the product of the 3 items.

A Therapeutic Footnote on Stability

As almost a footnote to the above analysis of stability one is tempted to point out its implications for therapeutic and rehabilitation techniques. It suggests a four-fold approach with the maladjusted in which one attempts:—

1 to adjust a man's job (both level and field) to his capacity and interest i.e. by some sort of selection procedure.

2 to overcome the effects of an inadequate group-cohesiveness by (a) giving him insight by some sort of individual and/or group psychotherapy (*the analytic aspect of psychotherapy*) and/or (b) by a job which makes fewer demands on his weaker qualities.

3 to raise his morale—after (1) and (2)—(a) by giving him opportunities of progressive and successful achievement—possibly by graduated participation in group projects—over a period: (b) by systematic but selective encouragement and appreciation over that period. This phase constitutes *the integrative aspect of psychotherapy*.

4 to augment his available energy by all the resources and armamentaria of physical and general medicine i.e. planned but not continuous sedation, re-creative holidays and new counterbalancing interests, appropriate exercise or instruction in muscular relaxation, etc., etc.

THE ORDER OF PROCEDURE

Beginning the Interview

One's first aim is to get the candidate talking freely: to project *his* personality and efface one's own. While it may be necessary to allow stress and tension to accumulate at various phases in the interview, one does not ordinarily do so at its beginning without special reason.

The 7–8 minute preliminary group-talk given by the psychiatrist on D1 produces a de-tensing effect which seems to save about 15 minutes in each interview: a considerable saving of time and sparing of emotional energy in bulk-interviewing.

The easiest "interview-opener" is to point to the ash-tray and say "do smoke if you wish". If he talks straight away—follow: if not, begin with an interview topic suggested by his Pointers i.e. some unusual interest, experience, viewpoint or statement; or with a stock opening question. One's own practice varied considerably with one's spontaneous mood or desire to experiment. It might be "what do you hope to do or be, eventually?" If no answer, after a pause, then "say, in 20 years' time?"

The direction of discussion in the next 3 phases is from the known to the unknown, the elicited to the spontaneous, the factual to the projective, from conscious elements to elements determined subconsciously; from queries about him to their specific answers.

Phase 1: The Factual Phase: Confirm and Complete the Facts.

The factual picture must be completed first. Most of it will have been analysed in a good Pointer: and it is poor tactics—and wasted time—to ask him to confirm what you already know and have no reason to doubt. One should quickly focus on what may have been omitted or about which one needs to know more: on apparent discrepancies, inconsistencies or lacunae in the biography.

This phase will be concerned largely with checking up on his level in the light of record, education and experience; with his social activities and group-cohesiveness; with his health record and the noting of any periodic recurrence of psychosomatic symptoms that may suggest a lessened stability.

Even in this factual phase one keeps the stream flowing fluidly and spontaneously: the candidate is encouraged to control it increasingly in his own direction: interstitial questions are interposed as lightly and delicately as possible: indicatively rather than interrogatively.

Phase 2: The Elicited Projective Phase: Explore his Range of Interests.

Using the known and the factual of Phase 1 as a diving point into the unknown and the projective, the candidate is continuously and gently manoeuvred into such spontaneity as he is capable of: one offers him the reins and lets him go where he wants to: the emphasis is shifted—unless the interview is too short or the candidate too "sticky"—from interviewer to interviewed.

Usually one will range over a number of fields of interest and evoke a projective reaction in each before letting the candidate settle down into those of dominant significance to him. A classification of these fields has been suggested in Chapter VIII in reference to the Interests Questionnaire. One quickly lists a variety of fields of interest: art, literature, music, current affairs, social and political matters, religion, philosophy, technical interests, science, sport, etc.: and gives him the opportunity to indicate whether his interest in each is great, slight or non-existent.

To plunge him quickly and easily into these fields, one finds the "projective" question more effective than the "yes or no" question. It acts as a trigger-release to his imagination: and encourages him to "free-associate", to "fan-out" into a particular field of interest. The projective question aims to get—not a specific answer, but—a characteristic response: a pointer to his attitudes and ideologies.

Examples are quoted on page 64. Here are more: some more suitable for the interview than the written test:—

> Whenever you feel tired or jaded, what is it gives you the greatest feeling of composure and relaxation?
> What game or sport are you best at? Do you enjoy most? Do you enjoy watching most? Do you wish you had taken up in the past? Would you take up now if you had unlimited opportunity?
> Your favourite character (living, historical or in fiction)? Favourite heroine? Favourite gramophone records? Pet aversions? etc.
> If you had all the money you wanted, what would you do for *pleasure*—as distinct from work?

With a flexible ever-changing repertoire of itemised systematically selected projective questions of this type, one can cover most large fields of interest in little time. Needless to say, one does not machine-gun him with questions: comment and interjection, question and response should so intertwine and balance each other that he feels himself increasingly guiding the flow and certainly not a passive target to be "shot at". The interviewer is sensed as intensely interested rather than intensely active.

In whatever field his response is positive, one follows it up in greater detail: given an interest in literature or music, one goes on to discuss authors or composers, etc. Sooner or later—after a preliminary exploration which indicates the width or narrowness of his range—one allows him to settle into a topic nearer his heart, about which he feels strongly and may be encouraged to talk spontaneously. There can hardly be an individual who has not one topic· he will talk freely about: sport, watching sport, reading about it, making things, listening to good music, reading, religion, scouting, etc., etc. The cluster of his interests may suggest he is predominately people-minded, thing-minded, idea-minded, or muscle-minded.

One tries to get him—so far as he is capable of it—into the habit of "free-associating" in the manner of the patient undergoing psychotherapy. Questions and interjections become shorter and less frequent: gaps and pauses widen out into which his spontaneous phantasy may flow. Once he sinks into a subject he likes—at whatever the phase—he is given the reins.

One notes not only the degree of spontaneity he is able to achieve but also the time and effort required to induce it: the crust of inhibition may be thin and due to superficial shyness; or thick and due to deep-seated factors which may not easily be influenced by training.

Phase 3: *The Spontaneous Projective Phase: Revealing the True Man.*

One's real aim is achieved when the candidate loses himself in his topic: is visibly attempting to clarify and formulate his views and attitudes—to himself as well as to you: and is, in effect, thinking aloud in your presence.

When achieved, this is a most satisfying experience for both: the candidate is especially grateful and this constitutes the most effective and natural way of "sealing" the interview. But it cannot always, or even often, be achieved. It requires time ($\frac{3}{4}$–$1\frac{1}{2}$ hours) and is never reached in less than 30 minutes, even under optimum conditions. With candidates who are very inhibited or "sticky", or who do not take to you, it may be quite impossible.

When the interview comes to a close, you are in a position—in conjunction with all you have learned before the interview—to make a reasonable estimate of the candidate's level, group-cohesive ability, morale, health, general stability and the sort of situations that may put strain on him. With luck and good management, you may have had actual samples (a) of the quality of his thinking in the interview, (b) of his group-cohesiveness in tasks and interview, (c) of his characteristic reaction to frustration in the impasses of the tasks or in the stressful pauses and topics of the interview.

Ending the Interview

The selection interview should never leave a man hurt, disconcerted or discouraged. He should go away happy: feeling, whatever the issue, that it has been interesting and even profitable, and that he has not been regarded as merely "job-fodder" to be "shot-at". Like every other social relationship, the interview should be two-way, prepared to give as well as get: more especially so because the medical psychologist's opportunity to probe deeply derives from his role and privilege as doctor and healer. Only by living up to the role and justifying the privilege can he hope to create and maintain rightful conditions for a useful contribution to selection.

Moreover the candidate has been through a gruelling test procedure: it seems only fair he should derive as reward some positive help from the obviously complete investigation into his personality. In the long run, vocational selection and vocational guidance are likely to merge into one and the same procedure: the welfare and interests of both employer and employee should be considered together and objectively. Until such time, it is important that the candidate should not resent any part of the procedure: if so, its value will diminish. Selection—like therapy—demands in the long run the co-operation of all concerned. You cannot select a man rightly—any more than you can treat him effectively—without his fullest co-operation. And you certainly cannot do either against his will.

One's own practice was to end the interview with what one called the "therapeutic hint": an offer of positive advice, help or information on any matter he cared to raise: apart of course from telling him the result of the Board which one did not then know and could not in any case divulge. One's penultimate question was "Is there anything you would like to tell or ask me?": then after a pause, "is there any advice or help or information of any kind I can give you?"

Often there is obvious stammer or admitted shyness where unasked one may offer constructive advice. Advice and re-assurance about a speech hesitation, shyness, stage-fright at interviews, minor phobias and physical ailments will always be appreciated. One will be consulted about minor personal problems, his suitability for certain jobs or careers, his strong points (which may be made clear if he is not sufficiently aware of them). One may advise him about admitted weaker points: how they may be helped by special studies, a change of social techniques or viewpoints, etc.: or mention books that may interest or help.

The introductory group-talk will have satisfied much of his curiosity about the psychological testing procedure. Sometimes enquiry about a particular part of the testing will reveal obvious doubts and anxieties. He should never be told his intelligence level except in very general terms but may be given a positive assurance as to what his abilities fit him for. It takes little effort and time to be constructively encouraging and to indicate one's good will: the accumulative effect of such an attitude on the prestige, goodwill and consequent effectiveness of a Selection Board can be considerable.

The general psychologist can adopt most of the techniques and principles here discussed provided he avoids any deep probing of anxiety-laden conflicts which his training has not prepared him to cope with; and can recognise the point where referral to a medical psychologist is advisable. The non-psychological interviewer should find assistance on a number of points; the evaluation of level, exploring the candidate's range of interests, estimating group-cohesiveness; and, from the notes below, on optimum interview conditions and reportage. He must be especially warned against uninformed and amateurish deep probing of emotional problems—so tempting for those with slight psychological training or experience—because of the upset and possible harm to the candidate as well as the likelihood of prejudicing the medical psychologist's ability to make his investigations. It is unfortunately too true that the amateur often rushes

G*

in where the medical psychologist would fear to tread. It has also happened that the latter has been discredited with the blame.

OPTIMUM CONDITIONS FOR THE INTERVIEW

DURATION

One's own experience is that a full psychiatric interview of this type requires 45–90 minutes: even under optimum conditions it will take 20–30 minutes to reach the spontaneous projection of phase 3.

With a well co-ordinated and conducted Board procedure, a much shorter interview of 20–30 minutes will be quite adequate for most cases: but not for all. About one in four of those interviewed (assuming that one interviews 25 per cent of the total batch) will need the longer period.

With very careful co-ordination with the rest of the test procedure, and if one has sufficient experience behind one, even a quite short 10–15 minute interview can be valuable: but as it will not provide one with that experience nor add to it, one is living on one's psychological capital.

LAY-OUT OF THE ROOM

Medical psychologists have their own preferences: some prefer to sit by the candidate: one's own feeling is that this is more likely to disconcert than reassure: as well as being a strain on one's neck. Sitting face to face across a lowish narrow table seems sufficiently intimate: the candidate in an easy chair. One's own preference is for an upright chair with arms to rest one's elbows: from which you can conveniently see your notes out of the corner of your eye and if necessary make a note, as if doodling.

Obviously conversation cannot flow if your eyes are glued to notes: yet with much—or even little—interviewing to do, one cannot hope to remember the details of each man's record. Any attempt to do so—so one found—killed one's spontaneity and there seemed no reason why one should try.

One's own solution—of which the "worksheets" described on page 53 are a simplified not so efficient version—was to represent the digested data about each group of 8–9 candidates on the two-paged conspectus of a moderate-sized notebook clipped to a millboard ($\frac{1}{4}$ page to each candidate). This was carried about with one and later kept for record.

In the rectangular area devoted to each candidate, the inmost section of about two inches square contained data from the Pointer: abbreviated, schematised and expressed numerically where possible: with coloured inks to make items stand out: different parts of the area were reserved for different activities and fields of interest: items were juxtaposed whose juxtaposition might automatically reveal a discrepancy and suggest a query (i.e. intelligence with schooling and educational standard: father's job with candidate's job or intended vocation, etc.). Unusual interests or experiences were marked to catch the eye.

Outside this square was a section for observations, GABI rank-ratings, facial profiles, nicknames, "verbatim samples" of conversation, etc. The third section on the margin of the page was for the first draft of one's pen-picture report. These 8 areas were numbered clockwise from 1 to 8 on the double page: for convenience in observing group discussions etc.

By glancing at this conspectus before the candidate entered the room, one noted interview topics and queries for special investigation. A casual glance at any time out of the corner of one's eye brought each point to mind without interrupting the flow of the interview. The full dossier was at hand if required. Ordinarily one made no notes but if one felt a verbatim remark might be forgotten, it was scribbled—as if doodling—on a blotter or scrap of paper and later transferred to one's notebook.

Good interviewing requires an unusual combination of spontaneity and precision which can in any volume be very stressful. For bulk interviewing one cannot dispense with techniques of this kind to give one the sense of security and control that comes from easy availability of all the data. They enable one to maintain a face-to-face relationship unbroken by distracting referrals to one's notes. Without that, one could not hope to achieve the third phase of the interview here described.

LIGHTING

Use of the light illuminates the quality of the interviewer: placing his "victim" in the light and himself in the shadow reveals sufficiently clearly that selection is not his métier. This is the technique of domination and intimidation: it reveals a sense of insecurity and a desire to impress: its intent is to project one's own personality, not that of the interviewee.

The interviewer is already—by virtue of his function—in a

privileged position which tends to create a "psychological distance": he must strive to minimise that gap if he is to get the candidate to project his natural personality. To increase the psychological distance by projecting and magnifying his own personality is a sufficiently clear revelation of psychological obtuseness and incapacity to de-tense the candidate. It will be interpreted—and rightly so—as a sort of "third degree".

It might occasionally be useful to adopt a therapeutic technique i.e. to put the candidate in the shadow and oneself in the light under inspection until he has gained confidence. But on the whole, the situation need not arise and it is best to sit near a window where features and expression are easily visible in both: and the relationship is open, frank and co-operative.

REPORTAGE

Quite early one discovers that impressions not noted immediately after the interview become hopelessly muddled. A personality must be described the moment it is savoured if one's pen-picture is to have any freshness. One's own practice was to scribble a first draft as the candidate left the room; and later to dictate 3 or 4 reports in one session. It can of course always be qualified by additional remarks.

Three Elements of Reportage for the Final Board

WOSB reportage on each candidate consists of 3 elements entered on a Profile Proforma (Appendix C) for use at the Final Board.

These elements are:—

1 The Background Summary (prepared from the Pointer material):

2 A profile of 17 items, rated in terms of a 5-point rating and with annotations:

3 A pen-picture, or summing up.

The Background Summary, plus the annotated profiles and pen-pictures of each individual observer for comparison, provide a very full reportage for the Final Board.

The Pen-picture

The pen-picture supplements the Background Summary and the annotated Profile and therefore need not be long. As no number of profile items can hope to cover the entire field of personality, it completes the picture, sums it up and incidentally notes the differentiae which make the candidate stand out as an individual.

The sort of headings one found oneself using at first are given below: they are of course purely personal. A sample pen-picture—invented to exemplify these headings—is given.

The Headings

A—his TYPE: physique, intelligence, regional type i.e. Yorkshire-man, etc.: *what sort of man* is he? with what sort of qualities? advantages? disadvantages? etc.

B—his BACKGROUND: socio-economic status, home happy or broken? etc.: *where does he come from?*

C—his PATTERN.

    1 *what is his specific aim or ambition?* i.e. what type of security does he seek (*qv.* Spranger, p. 64)?

    2 *what is his leitmotif or way of achieving this aim,* i.e. by work, social effort, opportunism, drifting, etc.?

    3 *how mature is this ambition or leitmotif and to what extent is his mode of attempting it objective, compensatory or evasive?*

D—his ACHIEVEMENT.

    what has been his development up to date in relation to his opportunities?

E—his SUITABILITY and PROGNOSIS and one's pre-Final-Board grading:

    how likely is he to adapt to the field and level for which he is being considered?

A Sample Pen-picture Analysed

TYPE, physical, mental, social, regional.	A red-haired Glaswegian student—short (5 ft. 2 ins.), be-spectacled, impetuous, and with a great deal of drive (not necessarily well-controlled)—
BACKGROUND	he comes from poor artisan stock (his father a dockyard labourer) and is an only child.
PATTERN	His high intelligence (OIR 9)—combined with a sense of inferiority deriving from his shortness, his myopia and his social background—seems to have led to a strong compensatory trend and a considerable ambition to shine academically.

ACHIEVEMENT   He has taken full advantage of every educational opportunity: by winning scholarships he has gained his Matriculation and a scholarship to the University where he hopes eventually to graduate in civil engineering.

PATTERN (*contd.*)   This he regards as an avenue of escape from the sort of life his father led. This urge and ambition does not come from his family but they are not opposed to it and are very proud of him.

PROGNOSIS and SUITABILITY   The hard work entailed has—despite his high intelligence—compelled him to force the pace and to drive himself: though he has managed to become a fair athlete, his social activities have been limited and he is still somewhat inhibited and shy: perhaps slightly egocentric, but fundamentally friendly and co-operative. He is strongly identified with the role of officer—or perhaps with the idea of officership—and has a strong sense of duty: though his sense of responsibility for the group is—because of inexperience and some degree of self-centredness—not very great. His tendency to drive himself will diminish his stability slightly but his social immaturity should diminish rapidly with training.

Provided he is otherwise suitable from the military viewpoint, he should eventually function adequately on about D level (i.e. just below average officer level) after training at OCTU.

In writing selection reports, derogatory remarks or "wise-cracks" at the expense of the candidate should never be committed to paper. It is especially inadvisable to emphasise personal reactions or private values: or to use such phrases as:—

I am (not) impressed.

He is *the right* (*wrong*) *type*, etc.

Remarks which imply comparison with oneself or an arbitrary

norm determined by oneself as to what is "the right type"—rather than an estimate of the man's capacities in relation to the job—are not conducive to an objective attitude and to the attitude of humility which befits those who approach the responsibility of determining the careers and functions of others. Especially so where one must objectively help to choose men for jobs for which one may not or need not oneself be suitable—or ever have been: which is of course inevitable if the variety of fields is as great as the number of Arms in the Army: or, for that matter, the possibilities in any major field like medicine, science, teaching, etc.

There is no reason why the psychological observer should not introduce—occasionally, gradually, relevantly and in reference to specific instances—words of psychological or psychiatric technical jargon in his reports. Indeed there is every reason why members of a team doing a psychological job should know more about psychological matters than, say, the man in the street. They are presumably selected as having some psychological flair and it is as much their duty to keep informed on psychological matters relevant to their job as it is the duty of the professional psychologist or psychiatrist to keep informed about the "job-analysis" aspect of selection. Each should give and accept guidance from the other.

Such words are best introduced when the Board has reached the stage of being able to appreciate their significance and use them fruitfully: they should not be permitted in the written reports of non-psychological members. But the cost of precision in their use is vigilance: without continuous guidance, abuses will inevitably occur: the over-anxious shy lad or the occasional hypomanic type will be labelled "schizoid": the word "immature" will cover everything from inexperience in a regional or fashionable code of manners to an obesity associated with endocrine deficiency.

CHAPTER XV

THE INTERIM GRADING SLIP OR SECOND INTERPHASE SCREEN

A *multum in parvo* screening device—initiated at 5 WOSB—was the Interim Grading Slip (IGS) which linked Phases 2 and 3: this helped to focus the full volume of the observer team's powers of observation on an ever-dwindling area of enquiry.

It was merely a slip of paper with 3 parallel columns (Appendix D) in which were entered the provisional gradings of team-leader, PSO and psychiatrist on the evidence available up to the end of Phase 2. One's own suggestion is that it might be entered here, in the Query Conference and early in the Final Board in terms of the GABI rank-rating which one found a particularly useful scale for both tests and interviews: a 4-point rating should be adequate for predictive estimates of this kind.

In a group of 8, there would on an average be discrepant opinions about one or two (their numbers might conveniently be starred on the IGS) and these one noted and discussed informally before the Final Exercise. One could then focus attention on them, and on the one or two residual queries about them. The rest one saw out of the corner of one's eye and usually confirmed the opinions shared by the team: only rarely was a reversal of shared opinion necessary.

This slip superseded—and was infinitely more convenient than—a bulletin board used in early WOSB practice, which presented the intelligence levels, provisional Spectrum or other ratings derived from the paper screening, the provisional gradings of each observer at the end of Phase 2, etc. The information about intelligence was later supplied in the much more detailed Background Summary and in the worksheets for use in the field: impressions and queries from the paper screening were made available in a more live and creative form in the free discussion of the Query Conference: the screening of gradings pooled after Phase 2 was more conveniently presented in the more mobile IGS.

The IGS is useful in several ways:—

1 As already suggested, it focusses and converges the full collective observing power of the team on a few queries about

a few candidates. The QC has raised queries which Phase 2 has attempted to answer: the IGS pools and compares these answers and from their discrepancies and residual doubts raises residual queries for Phase 3.

2 It compels the team to pool resources and work co-operatively and so leads to collective thinking of the most effective kind. In this way there will be less need for the Final Board to resolve wide discrepancies (a) by voting, in which numbers are decisive or (b) by debate, in which verbal arguments—presented too late for checking by test or experiment—may be decisive.

3 While encouraging collective thinking, it none the less illuminates the personal equation of each observer: indicates his trends, experience and flair: permits each to gauge—and so allow for—the quality of every other contribution: and indicates to the president the extent to which—in his judicial capacity— he should weight each opinion. No team can ever consist of members whose judgements are of equal value: there will always be weaker and stronger, more experienced and less, beginners and veterans. The IGS, in conjunction with the QC and Final Board, clarifies each observer's personal equation: is also a check on the judgements of each without in any way inhibiting these judgements. Indeed it trains by giving insight into such bias or deficiency as needs correction.

A fourth way in which the IGS might be made useful is by comparing and relating the recorded ratings at this stage with subsequent ratings after training i.e. at OCTU, or on the job. Between the IGS and the Final Board ratings, some convergence of opinion occurs: and to relate both these ratings statistically with subsequent ratings should throw some light on the contributions of individual observers.

CHAPTER XVI

RESOLUTION OF DISCREPANCIES AND CONFIRMATION: THE FINAL EXERCISE

In the Final Exercise (FE) one has one's last look at the candidates in action. Phase 1 has raised queries: Phase 2 has tried to resolve them and has come to fairly firm conclusions about most candidates. Such residual queries as remain have been called to one's attention by the IGS: and the FE provides the opportunity of resolving one's last doubts about one or two query candidates while casting a confirmatory glance at the others.

The usual FE was a 45-minute leaderless group task with 1–3 obstacles: the most important was usually of a "wide entry" type with a large total area so that candidates were spread out, easily observed and all could participate. A preliminary "shake-down" obstacle was not now necessary. One could employ more stress than in previous tests and this peak in the stress-curve tended to force a solution of the residual discrepancies.

A "double-entry" obstacle could be especially useful at this stage: the obstacle is negotiated from both sides and perhaps two on the far side are given a rope or other material means of helping the group across the obstacle. With this compulsion to participate, this selective "putting the heat" on the query candidates, the task ceases to be a pure leaderless group but is intermediate between it and the Command Situation.

All the groups tested in the batch (2–4) worked on parallel courses converging on a common or similar goal: the incentive therefore was inter-group rivalry rather than the time bogey. One interesting experiment was with an X type of group task in which two parallel groups, after racing across their first obstacle separately, united to form a group of 16 who were required to co-operate in order to cross the second obstacle: they then diverged to race separately across the third obstacle. The special intention of the X task was to compare—at the second obstacle—the level of leadership in both groups and to observe the reactions of leaders in one group to challenge by those in the other. While interesting and valuable as an experiment, the additional complication of a 16-member group did not strike one as adding to the practical value of the task.

One important consideration about Phase 3 is that by this time the procedure has freed and relaxed both the tested group and the observer team. The whole group—including the in-hibited, the immature and the slow-starting—have opened up and some of them may only now begin to reveal their potentialities. The observer team have solved most of their problems, have now only one or two queries about one or two candidates and the initial tension of acute discriminative observation has relaxed into an easier mental set. The jigsaw falls into place to reveal the total picture. Should there be any major doubt, two screening possibilities—besides the FB—still remain:

a a candidate not yet referred to the psychiatrist may be interviewed by him after the FE.

b there is the further screening effect of the Judgment Test.

One has already indicated one's predilection (p. 147) for the Human Problems Session as a FE in which the candidate's social personality may be seen "in the round" for the last time. This would be especially valuable in selecting for managerial, administrative, executive and professional fields.

CHAPTER XVII

A SOCIOMETRIC CHECK-UP: THE TEST OF OBJECTIVE JUDGEMENT

TWO GERMINATING POINTS IN THE DEVELOPMENT OF LEADERSHIP-TESTING TECHNIQUES

WOSB stresses the importance of group-cohesiveness in leadership: and the two germinating points of the WOSB approach, in one's opinion, are:—

1 the projective techniques by which it attempts to project this group-cohesiveness (a) on paper in the projection battery; (b) in speech, in the Human Problems Session, the UGD, the second part of the Planning Project and the psychiatric interview; (c) in action, in leaderless group tasks;

2 the attempts—tentative as yet—to project, record and even measure group-cohesiveness and to some extent group-effectiveness in a sociometric test, i.e. the Test of Objective Judgement.

The sociometric approach derives from the fertile brain of J. L. Moreno (in "Who Shall Survive"). Its purpose was to express graphically and quantitatively the dynamics of group inter-relationships and how each member of a group felt towards every other member; to illuminate the reasons for choice and rejection; and to reveal the popular and unpopular members, the disruptive and the cohesive.

Sociometric techniques still require further careful development and a more critical apparatus of analysis and interpretation. But even the simple technique here described can—with skilled psychological supervision and interpretation—yield fruitful results, intensify the interest of the observers in group inter-relationships, and both stimulate—and act as check on—their powers of observation.

BRIEFING THE TEST

The Test of Objective Judgement (also termed Inter-candidate Rating) was the last test before the Final Board. The group had by now worked side by side for three days and candidates were asked to give an indication of their capacity for objective judgement by ranking the other members of their group according to (a) the ability to influence others as leader, (b) the ability to get on with others as friend. That is to say each candidate was to rank each of his group-members from 1 to 7, in the order in which he could work happily, (a) *under* him as leader or officer, (b) *with* him as pal or colleague. He was also asked to give reasons for his first and last choice as leader. A further technical improvement is discussed below.

The test must be briefed and conducted by someone who fully appreciates its nature and purpose. It has happened that tactless and even stupid briefing by someone who has not been adequately informed, has reflected itself in a resentment of the test as a form of "snooping". On the one or two occasions when this has occurred, it seemed fairly obvious that the attitude of the group clearly reflected misconceptions in the mind of the briefing officer, who cannot therefore have briefed it with any conviction. The test is of course no more "snooping" than is any enquiry into the fitness of a man to accept responsibility on a higher level where he will influence the well-being and happiness of others. The well-intentioned responsible man, seeking increase in responsibility, does not resent enquiry into his abilities and motivation. Moreover even an elementary appreciation of the test's purpose should make it clear that it is not a popularity test and that the candidates ranked high by a particular group are not necessarily the best in that group.

To obviate unskilled briefing, one devised a self-briefing proforma (Appendix B) which explains the test clearly and concisely. Supplementary oral briefing is always necessary but the self-briefing makes it more "fool-proof" and does incidentally indoctrinate the briefer, as well as persuade and educate the candidate and thus prevent unjustified suspicions.

The briefing emphasises the importance in any responsible leadership of being able to distinguish objectively between one's liking for a man and one's estimate of his fitness for a specific job. It points out that the only way open to WOSB of estimating his objectivity is by comparing *his* judgements of the group with which he has worked with those of the observer team.

Though one has seen the test well administered by those without psychological training, one has no doubt that—like the paper tests of the Projection Battery—it should be conducted by the psychological department. Without that it is not possible to envisage any further technical development of the test.

HOW THE RESULTS ARE EXPRESSED: THE L/F INDEX

In the simple analysis used at WOSB, the rankings received by each candidate from the other seven were added up (i.e. $3 + 5 + 4$ etc.): the candidate with the smallest total ranked highest or first and the rest in order: if 2 candidates scored an equal number, they were ranked as equivalent i.e. if after the third candidate, they would both rank as $4 =$ ("equal fourth") and the next candidate would be ranked as sixth.

Two rankings were obtained for each candidate: one as Leader, the other as Friend. If he ranked fifth as Leader and third as Friend, what one might call his L/F index, would be 5/3.

INTERPRETING AND USING THE TEST

The test may be used:—

A—as a *testing* procedure, i.e. measuring and estimating;

B—as a *screening* procedure, i.e. comparing measurements and estimates and noting discrepancies as a pointer to further consideration;

C—as a procedure for *training* the observer team.

A—Purely as a Test

As a test, it enables one to project on paper the group's re-actions to each other, from which one may estimate:—

1 each man's *relative acceptability to that particular group* (from his ranking as Friend),

2 each man's *relative dominance and/or effectiveness in that particular group* (from his ranking as Leader).

These two rankings give a first approximation to the man as judged by the group.

Acceptability, is not the same as group-cohesiveness though it will ordinarily contribute to it. A man may be acceptable because of a personal charm which binds the group to himself but not to each other or to the group purpose or common advantage; another may be effectively group-cohesive without adding much to his acceptability. There is probably a considerable correlation between the two; and even acceptability *per se* does add to the collective warmth of the group.

B—As a Screening Procedure

Much more can be derived from the screening effect of comparing:—

  a the judgements of the observer team (preferably in a team
    GABI rank-rating of the FE), of the group and of its
    individual members:

  b each candidate's ratings as Leader and Friend (from his
    L/F index).

(*a*) throws light on the summated objectivity of the group
and the individual objectivity of its members: (*b*) throws additional light or confirmation on each man's group-cohesiveness
in that group.

The Objectivity of the Group's Summated Judgement

The group judgement is a summation of individual judgements
and *not* a collective judgement; it could only be the latter if the
group were to arrive at it after collective discussion. This judgement is not necessarily objective or good; and *the Judgement Test is
certainly not the measure of a man's personality by how the group vote for him.*
So naïf and incorrect an interpretation of the test must never be
allowed to rear its unscientific head. The group rankings give
some indication merely of that particular group's summated
reactions to each of its members; these reactions may be as foolish
or lacking in objectivity as any individual reaction.

A poor group will sometimes reject a quite outstanding
personality because of his very superiority, or because of his
complexity. A "dud" group of low OIR's will sometimes accept
—at any rate for the duration of a Board—the dominance
of a highly disruptive personality of superior intelligence. Groups
—like individuals, possibly more so—may be swayed decisively
and wrongly by the "halo" of combatant, overseas or Commando
Service; by seniority, NCO rank, etc., etc.

A comparison of the group rankings with the team's opinions
or rank-rating will usually confirm the general quality of the
group. Every major discrepancy between the judgement of the
group and that of the team about a particular candidate—one's
own estimate is that this will occur about once in every two
groups—should be specially considered and its reason resolved
so far as possible.

This is the sort of thing that happens. A candidate who seems,
to the observer team, pleasant and acceptable in every way is
unexpectedly rejected by the group and rated low as a friend.
This may indicate the dislike of an inferior group for a very
superior and complex individual. But it may also indicate—and

this is why it is so important to interpret and resolve such discrepancies—that the candidate has some vice more generally exhibited to a colleague or subordinate than to a superior in rank, which the procedure has not succeeded in projecting. Snobbishness perhaps, a tendency to toady, to disregard those who seem inferior or are handicapped, a fundamental selfishness or lack of warmth, etc.

Just as often, a candidate who strikes the team as insipid and colourless is rated high as a friend; possibly because of a quiet warm consistent friendliness by which he is able to establish contact with individual members individually, and is able to build up an atmosphere which may not be so evident when functioning on a collective job where his actual functional contribution may be moderate or low.

If the testing procedure has been good, the observations accurate and their interpretations correct, the observer team will be able to appreciate the reason for the group's discrepant opinions. By this screening of team and group opinion, the team is able to confirm its findings, check the occasional point it has missed and add precision to its judgements.

Just as one must learn—and allow for—the personal equation in the judgements of individuals, so one must learn—and allow for—the "group equation" when evaluating the group's rankings of its members.

The Objectivity of the Candidate

A really good candidate will give rankings which are consistently objective, if one makes allowance for relative inexperience and chronological immaturity. The ranking of the best candidate in a group will often provide the best reflex of the effect of each candidate on that group. In difficult groups—especially if borderline or poor—this ranking may contribute towards the resolving of doubtful issues.

A candidate who seems adequate or is considered borderline may reveal his poor judgement and appreciation of human values by his rankings of the group; and by the qualities which he indicates as important and presumably respects. Indeed each candidate reveals much of his personality and motivation by the choices he makes, the qualities he respects or dislikes and the reasons he gives for his choices.

Discrepancy in the L/F Index

The second screening comparison suggested is that between a candidate's ratings as Leader and Friend; as indicated by his L/F index. If he rates much lower as Friend than as Leader, this suggests a deficiency in group-cohesiveness; if much higher, it suggests a reserve of acceptability which may carry him further than a more gifted man lacking in this respect.

An L/F index of 1/8 would suggest a brittle leadership based perhaps on outstanding ability and dominance; but with little appreciation of the human factor to maintain that leadership against the depreciation of stress and time.

An index of 5/1 would suggest a man whose acceptability would reinforce such ability as he has. If his ability reaches the required minimal level for a certain field, one must consider—though he be lacking in some respects—whether this acceptability and its stabilising effect would not enable him to function adequately.

This index will either confirm or modify the general picture of the candidate. In a percentage of cases, it may contribute the critical evidence.

C—As an Aid to Training the Observer Team

By inducing observers to try to understand the reasons for unusual choices, antipathies, sub-groupings and group inter-relationships generally, the Judgement Test leads them to a wider and more sensitive appreciation of human beings and human relationships. One found that when the proformas and tabulated results were produced immediately before a Final Board, they were snatched up and read with as much avidity as any exciting news sheet. The test is also a check on the quality of the observations and raises discrepancies whose solving should lead to better decisions and improved judgement.

The self-briefing proforma is a continuous explicit reminder of the nature of objectivity and the need for it in their own judgements: it usually convinces candidates that they have had, not only an interesting experience but also a valuable lesson.

FURTHER DEVELOPMENT OF THE SOCIOMETRIC APPROACH

While the relatively simple undifferentiated technique here described can be extremely useful in many ways, the possibilities of future development are considerable. Each candidate in a group of 8, has 7 choices to make in each ranking, i.e. 14 choices in all. A simple technical improvement—which one has not so far had an opportunity to test—is incorporated in para. 5 of Appendix B. It should provide a more precise method of noting and analysing degrees of acceptance or rejection and constitutes a 3-point rank-rating of the GABI type. The next need is for a critical apparatus of analysis: such as the statistician may be able to supply.

Moreno and his co-workers—notably H. H. Jennings in "Leadership and Isolation", 1943—have investigated the mutual acceptances, mutual rejections and incompatible pairs (where one accepts the other but is rejected by him) that occur in groups who live together. Their methods have revealed those who are a focus of attraction or rejection in the group as well as those who have no effect at all. In short, they seem to have revealed the group-cohesive, group-disruptive and isolate types of personality and to have thrown light on some causes of both disintegrative and integrative sub-groupings and tendencies in the group.

Whereas Moreno and his co-workers seem to have investigated the social consequences of such types, it may be that the study of group dynamics in stressful situations where behaviour is fore-shortened and intensified may require modified techniques. It should however become increasingly possible to reveal—and measure—such types as MATCOP, IMAG and IMDEP; to differentiate between group-cohesive, group-disruptive and isolate patterns of behaviour; to evaluate more precisely the acceptability, dominance and objectivity of the members of a group; and possibly some of the other signs and roles considered in Chapter XIV. Here at any rate is a first attempt to express group behaviour and motivation in quantitative terms.

SOME AUXILIARY ENQUIRIES THAT MAY ACCOMPANY THE TEST

The second page of the self-briefing proforma included some additional questions to the candidate. These had nothing to do with the sociometric test; but as the testing procedure was now ending, it seemed a useful opportunity to obtain his reactions to the procedure, the WOSB and his own performance.

In question A he is asked to discuss his performance and factors that may have influenced it. In an attempt to justify or excuse himself at this stage, he may give important clues as to his *capacity for objective self-estimate*. These may be compared with his self-description in the Projection Battery, with his actual performance as judged by the observer team in a GABI rank-rating, with the group ranking of him, etc.

The other questions act usefully *as an emotional outlet*. They enable candidates to vent their petty grouses, complaints and resentments; to "seal" the testing procedure and sweeten their attitude to the selection board; and generally they help maintain the prestige, goodwill and future effectiveness of the Board with candidates to come.

They had more specific effects. They constituted a bi-weekly "Gallup Poll", a taking of the temperature of the candidate population, a sampling of its emotional climate and its emotional transference to the WOSB. As men and conditions change continuously on a selection board, this provided a most useful *check*—for the use of the President and board generally—*on the smooth administrative running of the board:* on the full availability of sleeping, eating, toilet, transport and other amenities. It enabled a board to maintain a high and improving standard in its reception and de-tensing techniques, etc. and provided it with points for formal or informal discussion with candidates. In short, it helped the board to apply stress where the procedure demanded it; and to remove it where it was not required.

FINAL AND GENERAL PROCEDURES

CHAPTER XVIII

THE FINAL BOARD AS THE LAST SCREEN

A—SOME THEORETICAL CONCEPTS ABOUT FINAL BOARD PROCEDURE

The Final Board as the Last Screen which helps Team Opinion to Converge

The Final Board is the last and ultimate screen.

"Testing" is the evaluation of observed performance level in tasks both social and functional: "screening" is any analysis of such evaluations as will result in a narrowing of the field of enquiry. To put it in another way. Testing is asking the right question to get the right answer. The appropriate task is the question, the performance level evaluated is the answer. Screening is a comparison of the answers to find out which are shared (and possibly correct) and which are not shared (and therefore in need of further investigation).

Residual queries left after a screening may be referred to another testing phase; or—where opinion has converged sufficiently—finally resolved by discussion as in the Final Board procedure: rather in the way that the pattern of a nearly completed jigsaw puzzle helps to point a place for the last few missing pieces.

The Final Board as a Gestalt Technique

In terms of Gestalt psychology, there are 3 phases in WOSB Final Board procedure:—

a a differentiation or "breaking-down" of the general picture or Gestalt into its component parts:

b an analysis of these parts with a view to clarifying those doubtful, obscure or about which there is discrepant opinion.

c a re-integration or "building-up" again of these parts into a new and clarified Gestalt.

These phases constitute a sort of Gestalt "calculus" of differentiation and re-integration and roughly correspond to 3 practical procedures which we will call (1) vertical screening, (2) lateral screening and (3) weighting.

In *vertical screening*, the general picture or Gestalt of the personality is broken down in a psychological profile into 17 items listed vertically below each other on the Profile Proforma and on the Profile blackboard on which individual and team gradings are chalked at the actual Final Board.

Vertical screening—as carried out by the President—consists of looking down the profile and picking out the two or three critical query items in each case: including those originally queried and those about which there is still discrepant opinion.

Lateral screening—as carried out by the President—consists of (a) picking out discrepancies in individual gradings of each profile-item; (b) presenting these for discussion to be resolved; (c) calling attention to the extent that general and specialist contributions of each observer to that item should be weighted. This lateral screening should lead naturally to a team grading of the item.

Whereas vertical screening deals with the vertical co-ordinate of *profile-item* and lateral screening deals with the lateral co-ordinate of *gradings of that item*, the third procedure of "weighting" deals with each observer's *global grading of the candidate* as a whole.

An element of weighting has already been considered in the lateral screening. In co-ordinating the global gradings of observers into a team grading, the President must weight each global grading as influenced by the age, experience, ability, objectivity and specialist experience of the observer. The composite, or rather product, of these weighted global gradings should lead to a truer estimate of the candidate and of the team's collective opinion of him.

The Final Board as a Technique of Collective Thinking

A collective effort of this kind polarises the team socially and functionally.

Socially, participation—even mere juxtaposition—in a common task is a powerful energiser and stimulates one to do with others what one might not bother to do by oneself.

Functionally, the specialist and general opinions of the team are polarised: firstly, by a selective referral of certain profile-items to certain observers: secondly, by a selective weighting of these specialist opinions before relating them to the opinions of the team in their non-specialist capacity. In this way an organic welding of everyone's general and specialist opinions results.

If in addition, the freest possible discussion is encouraged before the team-grading of each item and the final global team-grading of each candidate, a firm collective opinion is likely to result. The President is then in a position to use his vested authority to implement on his level what is in essence a collective decision.

This procedure, carried out at its best (as one has seen it), seems prototypic of collective thinking on its highest level.

B—THE CONSTITUTION OF THE BOARD

Up to late 1945, the President and Deputy President had equivalent functions: each interviewed one half of the batch and presided over one half of the Final Board. From this date, the President's function became entirely judicial: Deputy President and SPSO now performed equivalent functions and were termed Team-leaders: each interviewed one half of the batch. A third change will be discussed below.

Though theoretically the second procedure might seem to lead to greater objectivity, one preferred the first for several reasons.

The second procedure subtracts one from the number of PSOs available for testing and so diminishes the amount of work possible while adding to the expense. Depriving the President of actual participation in the testing—and some responsibility for evaluating it—seems in practice to lead to the temptation to superimpose unchecked judgements instead of evaluating the evidence, and to "interfere" with test procedure in default of other active participation. Moreover the *deus ex machina* contribution does not fit in with the modern trend towards team participation in any scientific approach.

The SPSO who, in his original function was able to teach, guide and supervise all of his PSOs, was then a key-man. Deprived of experience and practice in testing and sometimes appointed without previous experience as a PSO or in selection work, he was in no position to exercise any influence over his PSOs or to give them the instruction and guidance which they undoubtedly needed. Moreover, as an interviewer, his experience did not qualify him to be anything but a very pale imitation of a President.

Serious too is the lowering in status of the Deputy President and his deprival of the opportunity of presiding over part of a Board and of so becoming trained for Presidentship.

The natural ladder on the job-analysis side of the military selection board would seem to be: (1) PSO (chosen in the first instance as having aptitude for personnel selection): then, if promoted, (2) SPSO: after a period of regimental work, (3) Deputy Presidents might be appointed from among the ex-SPSOs: and some of these might go on to become (4) Presidents.

A third more serious change in the constitution of Boards occurred from early 1946 when psychiatrists and psychologists, as they ceased to be available, were gradually withdrawn. Without the availability of professional psychological help on the actual board, it seemed doubtful whether optimum scientific standards could be maintained: and certain, that further scientific development of testing procedure—still largely tentative and attempted only in a few fields—would be completely checked.

C—THE DATA AVAILABLE TO THE FINAL BOARD AND ITS PRESENTATION

In Chapter XIV it was pointed out that the reportage of each WOSB observer contained 3 elements which could conveniently be assembled on two sides of a foolscap proforma: (1) a Potted Biography or Background Summary, (2) a psychological profile of 17 items rated according to a 5-point rating, (3) a pen-picture report to complete the picture. A fourth element—available if required—was the psychological dossier containing the completed tests, questionnaires and projective material.

A fifth element, which should be available to increase the board's efficiency, encourage its growth and facilitate research, would be a Group Dossier to contain:—

1 The PSO's report on the behaviour and interactions of the group *as* a group:
2 the GABI rank-ratings of the Group Discussion, Progressive Group Task, Planning Project and Final Exercise (in a group reportage of the type described on page 49:
3 the raw material of the Sociometric Test and any analysis made of it.

D—HOW THE BOARD USES THE DATA

The Group Performance is Described

Before considering the candidate, it is useful to know about the group in whose context he has been observed: this is where

the group dossier would help.   The PSO describes in chronological order the group's behaviour, conflicts and sub-groupings:
how it has coped with its tasks, crises, impasses, difficult members,
etc.   A GABI rank-rating of the Basic Series and Final Exercise
would provide a useful statement of its quality and a peg for
discussion in detail.   Where the Sociometric Test has been
analysed, the psychologist or psychiatrist might be asked to
comment on the group's general interactions: details about
specific candidates are better discussed with the candidate.

The Candidate's Biography is Considered

As the Background Summary is an analysis of the candidate's record prepared by the Sjt-Testers, this would be a good
time to bring him "into the picture" by asking him to summarise
it and call attention to its highlights.   In practice, this was done
by the Team-leader.   From the biography were derived gradings
for the profile-items (1) Leadership Experience and (4) Educational Standard.

His Military Record is Noted

From this is obtained his grading on profile-item (2) Unit
Report.   This was considered at the Query Conference in order
to raise queries for investigation: it may now be re-considered
again by the Team-leader in the light of that investigation.
This will illuminate not only the candidate but also the quality
of the unit reporting on him.

The Team Profile is Worked Out

This phase is conducted by the President.

On a large blackboard are listed the 17 profile-items: opposite
each item are spaces for a 5-point rating of Good, Satisfactory,
Borderline, Weak or Very Weak: an assistant chalks the initial
of the observer (T for Team-leader, P for PSO, S for psychiatrist
or psychologist) in the appropriate space.

Where gradings correspond (are in the same space) a
vertical line is drawn through it.   With discrepant gradings, if
there is one dissident he is asked to state his reasons.   If each
grading is different, discussion follows: at first in the order of
PSO, Team-leader and psychiatrist, then spontaneously in no
set order.

Generally the team will agree on a common grading, through

which a vertical line is drawn. A member who cannot accept the team grading is allowed to "box" his grading (a circle or square is drawn round it) to record dissent for purposes of reference or research. Discussion revolves mainly round discrepant gradings. With the completion of the 17 team gradings, the team profile of the candidate now stands out.

Wherever one rates a candidate low on an item, one usually scribbles a few words of explanation in a column to the extreme right of one's proforma, opposite that item. It is also useful, wherever discrepancies reveal themselves in the course of the Final Board, to scribble at the time some words to explain and justify one's difference of opinion.

It is particularly important that every profile-item should have a clear operational definition which is readily available and often consulted.

The Reading of Pen-Picture Reports is Followed by a Final Discussion

These are read by PSO, Team-leader, then psychiatrist (whose report may explain aspects of the candidate's observed behaviour noted by the others).

Most discrepancies have already been resolved in working out the team profile. The President may ask observers to discuss, amplify, and finally clarify discrepant points in their reports.

Observer Opinions converge into a Collective Opinion

With a good board procedure and an effectively co-operating team, one hopes to find observer opinion converging and crystallising very naturally into a collective opinion which for the most part satisfies everybody. And sufficiently often, one does.

With the pooling of all the data, the total picture will not necessarily correspond with one's own view of part of that picture. The objective observer does not identify himself so rigidly with his own opinion as to regard a final team opinion which does not correspond with his own part opinion as an implicit challenge to the quality of his judgement.

One's own experience was that with a good team, however the final judgement differed from one's own opinion, one usually felt it to be right. Where one felt consistently that it was not so, either one was a poor team member or in a poor team.

H

Presidential Authority Implements that Collective Opinion

The President's function at the Final Board seems to be a two-fold one:—

a to use such experience, wisdom and forceful drive as he possesses to assist obstetrically in the formation of a sound collective opinion and decision:

b to use the rank and authority vested in him to implement this collective decision—to which he may have made a major contribution—on his own level of authority.

He should not regard the procedure as a voting matter in which his is the casting vote. For a President to insist on his absolute right to make the final judgment—even against the opinion of his team—is to insist on an outmoded and untrue conception of leadership.

On the one hand, to the extent that he aims to show true leadership by presenting himself as an exemplar of objective judgement, he will not rigidly identify his own predilections or opinions with the ultimate team decision.

On the other hand, though he was considered to be technically responsible for the final decision, one would suggest that the responsibility cannot justly or wisely be made to rest on him alone: it must be shared with the team, though his may be the major share. It has been suggested (page 141) that authority and responsibility are commensurate with function. Function on a higher level carries greater authority and more responsibility. In so far as selection by a Board is a collective function, no one on the Board can carry all of the authority or all of the responsibility. Any attempt to make him do so creates an overloaded and brittle individual leadership by domination, and is an abuse of vested authority.

E—GRADING THE CANDIDATE

The Grading Scale Used

The scale used was defined as follows. In any sample of 20 commissioned officers, the middle 8 are considered to be on average officer level i.e. on C level: the 4 above on B level, the 4 below on D level: the top 2 on AB level, the bottom 2 on DD level: the best officer in 100 on A level. As the A is seldom used, this is—along with the F or Fail grading—in effect a 6-point grading.

At a much later stage, only the gradings B, C, D and F were

used: in one's own experience, a 4-point grading is easier to manipulate and in predictive estimates of this kind is adequate for all practical and research purposes.

The Tendency to Down-grade

There was in WOSB practice a very definite tendency to down-grade. According to definition, B's should have been as frequent as D's (i.e. 1 in 5) and AB's as frequent as DD's (i.e. 1 in 10) yet D's and DD's were much more frequent than B's and AB's.

At one time one felt that this down-grading might be the reaction of an insecure Board against seeming too lenient: one has little doubt that this compensatory down-grading does play some part and that it is accompanied by a narrower range of gradings.

Sometimes the down-grading was rationalised as due to the deteriorating quality of the candidate entry as the war went on i.e. "scraping the barrel". Here too, one felt there might be confusion in failing to distinguish between the quality of a man's motivation and the quality of his abilities.

Some evidence however seems to be accumulating to suggest that officer levels do not distribute themselves symmetrically around the mean, but do in fact increase in frequency with the fall of level.

If this proves to be so, it does seem important that a scale more in accord with the actual distribution should be in use and that standard criteria and definitions should correspond with the nature of the material. Unless they do, the efficiency of grading is likely to be impaired.

Assuming a scale which is not a Procrustean bed—and one will have to be worked out—how then ensure more uniform standards and a juster distribution of gradings over the scale?

A 2-Phase Method of Grading

Ordinarily, each candidate was finally graded after pooling the relevant data.

What seemed a better method was in use at 15 WOSB, Leeds in 1944. All candidates were first graded as Pass or Fail (I prefer the terms Suitable or Unsuitable which merely indicate suitability for a specific field of activity and do not reflect on the candidate's suitability for other—possibly more important—fields).

At the end of the Board, all the Suitables in the batch were ranked—working from the best downwards—and given their final grading. This is in effect a rank-rating of the GABI type.

A first result of this 2-phase grading is a more even and juster distribution of gradings. Equally important is the fact that by compelling the entire team to attend the entire Final Board Session (PSOs ordinarily attended only the discussion of their own group: and Team-leaders the discussion of their own half of the batch) it enabled the President to establish and maintain common Board standards. Without such a combined session, Team-leaders and PSOs had no direct means of exchanging experiences, fertilising each other technically, nor of working out common standards: nor could PSOs learn from the SPSO where he happened to be a practising PSO.

Concomitant with this 2-phase grading, 15 WOSB used a 6-monthly histogram showing graphically the actual distribution of Final Board gradings in that period: on this was superimposed a histogram of the expected distribution according to the criteria laid down. A skew histogram, humped to the left for instance, would suggest that the Board was down-grading: a hump to the right that it was up-grading. This could also be carried out for the individual observers on the Board.

Unsuitable Candidates should be Classified in Terms of
Their Inadequacy

Experience with the Spectrum Rating suggests that while Suitables should be graded in terms of their likely level after training, Unsuitables might usefully be classified in terms of the type of inadequacy considered responsible for their unsuitability: and rated where possible in terms of levels below officer or leadership level.

The Spectrum Rating used by the Psychological Department does in effect combine a rating of level with a classification of the lower levels in terms of the types of inadequacy responsible for them. It would be improved if it were to discriminate more precisely than it does the levels below that of officer. Indigo A2 (NCO level) is the only attempt it makes in this direction. It would certainly be helpful—both to the candidate and the community—if those likely to be adequate on the various NCO, foreman or technician levels were so rated: so that they might be advised or helped towards their optimum functional level.

A classification of this sort may be useful for the following reasons:—

a Out of the working experience of any selection team, there will arise pragmatically a typology of inadequate individuals. The attempt to classify each case as it arises will test and clarify this typology and make it increasingly precise. It will also train selectors to raise appropriate, relevant and fruitful queries at the query stage of investigation.

b It will throw light on impediments to the realisation of potential leadership and consequently on the nature of leadership itself. In so doing, it will suggest how one may advise and help those who have failed: and those who will employ them.

c It will facilitate a detailed analysis and follow-up of rejected, as well as accepted, candidates. This should provide checks on—and aids to—board efficiency. It has already been used to relate Sjt-tester ratings with OCTU gradings.

Short-term Validation as an Aid to Training

The statistical implications of selection validation are discussed in Chapter xx by a statistical psychologist. A word here on validation as an aid to training.

WOSB standards have been checked by correlating the gradings of Boards and of individual Board members with gradings at OCTU after 4–9 months of intensive observation while training for officership. It is intended to carry out this comparison at 3-monthly intervals.

This, one might regard as a short-term validation because it does not yet grade the man's efficiency on the actual job. If after some months of such observation and training, he is graded as suitable, the likelihood is that WOSB was justified in regarding him as worthy of the opportunity of training. Which is perhaps as much as it might legitimately be expected to do. Other more cogent reasons for accepting the validity of this comparison are given in Chapter xx.

With such short-term validations—using suitable checks— it is becoming possible to determine the efficiency not only of Boards but also of their individual members: and in respect of specific types of candidate (for different Arms, from different schools or classes in the community, etc.). Under certain conditions (the systematic use of GABI rank-ratings, etc.), it should be possible to evaluate and validate the specific contribution of specific test procedures to Board gradings.

What seems of especial promise here is the possibility of using such a "resonance" of OCTU opinion back to WOSB not merely as a measure of efficiency but also as an aid to training the Board. A detailed routine 3-monthly analysis of the comparison should indicate tendencies, either in the Board or its members, to down-grade or up-grade: or to bias with specific types of candidate.

Knowing how one would have welcomed a periodic "resonance" and check of this kind on which to whet one's judgement, one feels that such short-term validations might constitute part of the routine training and guidance of a selection board. One gathers that this is now to become routine practice.

In any large-scale selection scheme, long-term validations in relation to efficiency on the actual job are also necessary. But while they may—or may not—provide a better validation of the Board, they cannot be of value for immediate training purposes.

F—THE PSYCHOLOGICAL PROFILE IN DETAIL

The 17 Profile-points

The purpose of the WOSB profile—with its 17 profile-points—was to induce observers to cover, if not all of the ground, at any rate a large part of it. The items were not exclusive categories. It was not intended that the final global grading should correspond with the shape of the profile: though, with increasing experience and an increasing agreement on common standards of rating, it would tend to.

Each item was rated on a 5-point rating of Good, Satisfactory, Borderline, Weak and Very Weak.

The items were as follows:—

1 LEADERSHIP EXPERIENCE i.e. in social and athletic clubs, societies and teams.

2 UNIT REPORT i.e. on behaviour and performance while in the Army.

3 OIR (Officer Intelligence Rating) in terms of the indices 1–10 described in Chapter VIII.

4 EDUCATIONAL SUITABILITY in terms of the indices 6–1 described on page 57.

5 PLANNING ABILITY.

6 PRACTICAL ABILITY.

7 ATHLETIC ABILITY.

8 LEVEL OF AIMS i.e. type of job and level of responsibility sought in life.

9 EFFECTIVENESS IN PURSUIT OF AIMS. This is partly an estimate of the success already achieved in relation to his opportunities: partly a predictive grading of the likelihood of his succeeding in his future aims.

10 MILITARY COMPATIBILITY. This might be interpreted as

   a his identification with the Army
   b his suitability for the Army *on officer level.*

Thus a regular soldier who had entered the Army as a boy and worked his way up to RSM might be graded Good according to (a) but Borderline according to (b). The second was the more usual interpretation. As indicated later in this chapter, one considers the first interpretation to be correct. The second anticipates the final global grading and results from confusing, and failing to distinguish, the concepts of field and level.

11 SENSE OF RESPONSIBILITY. The degree to which he is identified with the group's job, purpose and welfare. This is more than a sense of duty i.e. the degree to which he identifies himself with his own particular job and function within the group without reference to its relationship to the total group purpose.

12 SOCIAL INTEREST i.e. his intellectual awareness of the human problems of individuals and groups.

13 QUALITY OF PERSONAL RELATIONS i.e. his ability to bind the group to each other and to a common group purpose —to get them working harmoniously on a task.

14 RANGE OF PERSONAL RELATIONS i.e. his ability to get on with individuals of different types and levels (superiors in rank, colleagues, subordinates).

15 DOMINANCE i.e. his ability to impose his will on others.

16 LIVELINESS i.e. his ability to stimulate others.

17 STABILITY OF HEALTH. This is a global rating of his combined physical and mental health and stamina and the extent to which he is able to stand up to a reasonable degree of stress and to a reasonable variety of types of stress over reasonable periods of time and at reasonable tempos without breaking down.

Comments on Some of the Profile-points

LEVEL OF AIMS may be considered in two senses (a) in the absolute sense of the level of the job sought in life i.e. professional or officer level, highly skilled, unskilled, etc. (or in equivalent Army ranks—WO, Serjeant, Corporal, etc.): (b) in the relative sense of comparing the level aimed at with the socio-economic status of the home he comes from, i.e. a miner's son aiming to be an engineer would be rated high whereas a professor's son aiming at the same level, would be merely satisfactory.

The former was the sense usually adopted: the latter was better considered under "Effectiveness in Pursuit of Aims" (9).

A few profile items i.e. 1–4 are evaluations of past and present: most however—like 9, i.e. EFFECTIVENESS IN PURSUIT OF AIMS—are partly predictive in that they attempt to assess the candidate as he will be after a period of training.

As suggested, a SENSE OF RESPONSIBILITY (11) connotes a wider identification with the group than a sense of duty which confines itself to an identification with the job alone. The man with a sense of duty might be contented to carry out his orders to the letter even if he knew that a change of circumstances had rendered them senseless. Had he a sense of responsibility, he would have been sensitive to the changing needs and demands of the group purpose: and would have considered himself responsible for doing something about it. One might relate the level of a man's sense of responsibility to the size of the group with which it is identified.

Profile points 13 and 14 together constitute group-cohesiveness as defined and discussed in this book. The former includes the latter: the ability to bind a group does imply the ability to deal with the different types of people and the different functional levels to be found in every group.

About DOMINANCE (15), one does not feel so happy. WOSB experience emphasises the importance of the ability to influence and persuade and bind a group rather than to drive it: the type of behaviour commonly recognised as dominant is less likely to bind a group than ultimately and progressively to disrupt it. Elsewhere it has been suggested that the best type of leadership is likely to exist in inverse proportion to that form of crudely extroverted aggression which is ordinarily recognised as strong dominance.

In the profile, qualities present in high degree come under

the Good rating (to the extreme left of the 5-point rating): a high degree of dominance would—one suggests—indicate a poor rather than a good candidate: at any rate, one who was poor in the ability to influence the group happily.

True, it has been suggested that there is a good type of dominance—a persuasive type—as well as a bad type. But in view of the general connotation of the word (which may derive from its association with "domineering"), one feels it is best dropped as a profile-item.

In so far as it may imply "persuasiveness", that is already considered in items 13 and 14. In so far as one wishes to consider the capacity to take a strong line when that is indicated, better terms would be "Firmness" or "Capacity for Firmness" or "Self-assertiveness". In so far as firmness is acceptable to the group because it meets a real need, it might be rated Good: firmness which is dominant or disruptive might be rated Border-line or Weak.

With regard to LIVELINESS (16) there is a restless liveliness which is disturbing and an easy spontaneous liveliness which is stimulating. The term "Spontaneity" or "Spontaneous Liveli-ness" would distinguish the stimulating quality from the com-pulsive restlessness.

Ratings on STABILITY (17), are a matter for the medical psychologist. Some attempt should be made to establish common and equivalent standards which may be distributed over a scale: preferably a 4-point GABI one.

A grading of Very Weak by the medical psychologist should be regarded as a definite clinical diagnosis of serious instability and medical unfitness for the job: as definite as a down-grading of medical category.

In the matter of health—physical or mental—there must be a point where the authority of the physician becomes decisive: if there is to be an appeal, it should be to a higher medical authority. This rating should of course only be made where the certainty is such that it would be improper for the President— or any lay authority—to disregard it. To do so would be equiva-lent to ordering into the front line a soldier graded as of C category because of severe neurosis, or one requiring hospitalisation.

The rating of Weak should be used to indicate considerable risk of breakdown on officer level: a risk which might however be taken if the candidate's abilities are high or outstanding in

H*

relation to the job's requirements. Many of the best and most efficient people will be relatively unstable individuals who elect to function and work adventurously on levels above their optimum.

G—THE FUTURE OF THE PSYCHOLOGICAL PROFILE

The WOSB profile is a first tentative formulation of some of the major fields in human adjustment on leadership level. Its practical value was, and is, considerable: but the need for its further development is obvious enough; and the attempt should be both profitable and interesting.

In Chapter xiv, one has suggested a 3-fold clustering of items around the concepts of level, group-cohesiveness and stability. Some preliminary statistical comparisons of WOSB gradings with OCTU gradings seem to indicate the relative importance of items 3 (Intelligence), 4 (Educational Standard), 13 (Quality of Personal Relations and 14 (Range of Personal Relations): of these, the first two are related to level and the last two to group-cohesiveness.

The rating on Stability (17) cannot easily be correlated with officer careers: partly because the spread over the 5-point rating was slight but mainly because those with lower gradings were not likely to become officers. However, some work done by the author on officers who broke down psychiatrically after passing a WOSB reveals a significant correlation between these cases and a combination of relatively low intelligence and low educational standard.

In breaking down the Gestalt of the personality to permit of investigation, it would be useful to have a first differentiation into clusters such as these three, as a sort of half-way house before breaking down each cluster into its component items. Similarly, in integrating one's findings after investigation on the way back, one would appreciate a half-way clustering of one's items into these three larger related patterns.

A Suggested New Profile

If I were to draw up a new profile for practical or experimental purposes, this is the sort of profile I should begin with: the items to be defined as in Chapters xiii and xiv and rated on a 4-point GABI rating.

Record and Report

    1 RECORD OF SOCIAL PARTICIPATION AND RESPONSIBILITY.
I would prefer this to "Leadership Experience" which
it would of course include.

    2 REPORT (scholastic or vocational) on recent efficiency,
social "contact", nature of general and special interests,
force of character, any weak or undeveloped traits, etc.

The Level Cluster

    3 OIR.

    4 ES.

    5 ASPIRED LEVEL for "Level of Aims".

    6 COMMENSURATE EFFECTIVENESS for "Effectiveness in pursuit
of aims".

    7 IDENTIFICATION WITH THE FIELD for "Military Com-
patibility".,

    8 PLANNING ABILITY, i.e. the extent to which the candidate
uses his OIR and ES effectively in the test procedures.

    9 WIDTH OF INTERESTS (social, technical, cultural, etc.): as
defined in "Sampling the Quality of a Man's Thinking"
in Chapter XIV.

The Group-cohesiveness Cluster

    10 WARM SPONTANEITY: to replace "Liveliness" and "Range
of Personal Relations".

    11 OBJECTIVITY or the ability to distinguish and relate the
interests of Group and Self. This is related to the "Self-
estimated Level": and along with "Identification, etc."
(7) with "Sense of Responsibility".

    12 CAPACITY FOR FIRMNESS or the ability to control group-
disruptive tendencies in the individual or group: to
replace "Dominance".

    13 TACT or the ability to combine firmness with encourage-
ment and the raising of morale.

    14 ABILITY TO BRING OTHERS INTO THE PICTURE and to relate
them *emotionally* to the job: to replace "Quality of Personal Relations". This ability implies the existence of
"cooperativeness". It must be distinguished from
relating people *functionally* to the job (i.e. allocation)
which is considered under Planning Ability (8).

The Stability Cluster

15 STABILITY is best left as a single profile item but may usefully be considered by the medical psychologist under
4 sets of factors:—

a *Level factors:* the relationship between potential level
(*qv.* 3 and 4), actual level (*qv.* 6), aspired level (*qv.* 5),
required level (explicit in the job-analysis) and self-
estimated level (*qv.* 11).

b *Group-cohesiveness factors.* Four of the five signs described
in Chapter XIV are contained in this profile: the
fifth i.e. "cooperativeness" is implicit in (14).
Of the social roles described in Chapter XIII, three
are contained above: "empathy" is implicit in (10),
"encouragement" in (13).

c *Morale,* or one's proneness—as determined by one's
past experiences—to success or failure in the job.

d *Drive,* i.e. the availability of energy as determined by
physical and mental health and make-up. Drive in
this sense of the word must be clearly distinguished
from the re-direction and consequent availability of
energy for a special purpose that is determined by
the candidate's identification with the field (7);
and which derives *not* from his general make-up and
present health but from his attitude to the job.
Attitudes do of course strongly influence the availability of energy in specific directions: and as such
are important determinants of group-effectiveness.
It seems however more convenient to consider
attitudes—along with aptitudes—in the Level
Cluster.

This profile includes in some form or other all the signs of
superior adjustment and all the roles demanded by the job on
leadership level that are described and defined in Chapters XIII
and XIV. While one found these concepts of practical value in
observation, judgement and teaching, only clinical experimentation with statistical follow-up can indicate to what extent—singly
or in combination—they can be of value in a profile for general
use.

FINAL AND GENERAL PROCEDURES

CHAPTER XIX

THE FUNCTIONS OF THE PSYCHOLOGICAL DEPARTMENT

The Psychological Department was in the charge of the psychiatrist assisted by the psychologist. The latter, for most of the time, was not allowed to interview or function as a grading member of the Board. Both psychiatrist and psychologist co-operated in training and supervising the Sjt-Testers.

THE ROLE OF THE SJT-TESTER: BRINGING HIM "INTO THE PICTURE"

The Sjt-Tester was first employed to administer paper tests and prepare a Personality Pointer for the psychiatrist: later he was required to prepare from the biographical details, a Background Summary for the other members of the Board.

One felt this procedure to be unsatisfactory for the following reasons:—

a In analysing biographical and projective material, he was living on psychological capital and experience of which he had little or none.

b He was being deprived of the exceptional opportunities of acquiring, and adding to, his experience by observing groups under the experimentally controlled stress conditions provided by WOSB.

c As a "backroom boy", he never found himself "in the picture" with the rest of the team and had insufficient social or other incentive to give of his best.

Because of one's feeling that he must be treated as a junior psychologist, permission was obtained—mainly at 10 WOSB— to give him opportunities for observation. He was allowed to observe the group he was analysing in the Basic Series and Final Exercise: to participate in the various screens, i.e. Query Conference, Interim Grading, Judgement Test and Final Board: and to co-operate in tasks which contained a strong projective element i.e. choosing officer problems and stooge roles for the Human Problems Session.

He could now compare his interpretation of the paper screening with his observation of the group and so become more sensitive to paper pointers which he might otherwise have missed. He could also amplify or modify his original Personality Pointers so that full psychological reports—which were not merely pointers for the interview—could be made available on every candidate at the Final Board. He could also give a Spectrum Rating of the candidate in terms both of level and—if unsuitable—of his type of inadequacy.

This experiment became one's regular practice at 10 WOSB. It seemed more than justified by the very full psychological screening of the entire batch of candidates that it permitted: by the Sjt-Testers' continuously increasing skill, sustained enthusiasm, improved relations with all members of the Board and helpfulness to the psychiatrist. The latter had no doubt that it increased the volume, sureness, ease and value of his own contribution. Later scrutiny of a sample of these Spectrum Ratings in relation to subsequent OCTU gradings seemed to confirm their value and to justify this fuller use of the Sjt-Tester.

THE ROLE OF THE PSYCHOLOGIST

The psychologist was especially concerned with:—

a the administration, supervision and interpretation of group and individual intelligence tests and of paper screening generally:

b the evaluation of educational standards in relation to vocational requirements:

c the collection of data for graphic representation and Board validation:

d helping to maintain a scientific methodology in testing, observation and grading.

THE ROLE OF THE PSYCHIATRIST

The special contributions of the psychiatrist were:—

a to advise on *present* physical and mental *health:*

b to make a predictive estimate of the candidate's likely physical and mental stability on the higher level required:

he might be stable on OR level yet unstable on officer level:

c to make a predictive estimate of the candidate's future *development and likely social maturity*, after further training and experience.

d to teach, supervise, control and check *the interpretation of projective material*, written or otherwise (for which, only clinical experience derived from deep analytic therapy could qualify one):

e perhaps his main function was advisory and educational in that his specific reports and general advice should help the Board to become progressively aware of the "complex 25 per cent" of the candidates, the factors to be considered in their placement and when referral to the psychiatrist is indicated. Optimally, with the increase of this function, the number of referrals should decrease and those referred can be more intensively studied and reported on.

In respect of these five points he is the only member of the Board professionally qualified to give an opinion.

Even the young physician, untrained in the psychological approach, has an extensive experience of suffering mankind: of men and women taking stresses that are sometimes too much for them: the stress of illness, loss or threatened loss of dear ones, impending death, etc. The medical psychologist—by virtue of his special training and experience—has an even wider and deeper knowledge of these things.

He cannot help acquiring a flair for sensing the psychosomatic predispositions of people, the organs likely to crack up under strain, the early symptoms of breakdown in different types. Each man cracks up in his own way: one becomes a cardiopath, another a gastropath, another an arthropath, a frank hysteric or anxiety neurotic: stress may lead to a peptic ulcer, exophthalmic goitre, diabetes, migraine, asthma, eczema, angina pectoris, etc., etc.: the physician—more especially the medical psychologist—has the most intimate opportunity of becoming acquainted with the earliest psychosomatic and other pointers to failing morale.

His prestige and function as a healer give him privileged opportunities to learn about a man: it is not usual for people to approach the doctor in a bluffing attitude. So long as he remains the physician on a selection board—and there is every reason why he must—he is in a position to make special contributions because of this trust in him: one which he must never abuse.

We have already suggested that what the medical psychologist still lacks to redress the balance of his experience—in view of the increasingly constructive role in the community he is being called upon to play—is an extension of that experience to include a number of those who are adjusting to life on a very superior level.

THE ROLES OF PSYCHIATRIST AND PSYCHOLOGIST ARE NOT EQUIVALENT

The functions of psychiatrist and psychologist are complementary: never equivalent. They must never divide a batch of candidates into two equivalent and separate halves; but must co-operate in investigating the same field from different but complementary viewpoints.

A good psychiatrist working with a good psychologist should be more effective than two psychiatrists or two psychologists covering the same ground. A perfect combination would be that of psychiatrist, psychologist and statistician. One's own preference is for the *ad hoc* statistician on the spot rather than the *post hoc* statistician who intervenes *after* the data have been collected. One cannot help feeling that in the measurement of human qualities, the quantities and integers used are approximative and far from absolute: and that the modifying "values" of the men who measure, and of the measuring procedures and criteria they use, are best allowed for by the statistician who has had some participation in the actual experiment. This however is properly a topic for the next chapter.

WHO SHOULD BE IN CHARGE OF THE PSYCHOLOGICAL TEAM?

WOSB put the psychiatrist in charge because he was largely concerned with the initial experimentation upon which its technique was based; and because such psychiatrists as were available for the job were less inexperienced than the available psychologists.

The psychologist's training does not as yet provide clinical experience of interviewing men or observing human relationships under stress or under experimental conditions. The physician is compelled to study his raw material—the living patient—before he is allowed to go on to become even a medical laboratory scientist or statistician. The psychologist should not be deprived of a similar opportunity of studying his raw material, i.e. mankind and human relations—either in the interview situation, the experimental group or the specialised communities of workshop or factory—before he goes on to work in a narrower, more special, area of the field of human relations. This is not—as yet—readily available to him, though it must increasingly become so.

Where the function of a psychological team is therapeutic, i.e. in psychiatric clinics, one would expect the therapist responsible for treatment to be in charge. In a team primarily devoted to academic research, the academic psychologist might take charge.

In selection—where physical and mental and vocational suitability are being considered—there seems to be no special reason why either should be in charge. Their functions might well be regarded as equivalent: and their rank related to seniority and experience in their own field.

THE PSYCHOLOGICAL CONTRIBUTION AS A COLLECTIVE EFFORT

A feature which helped to bind and train the psychological team at 10 WOSB—as well as being an expression of its cohesion and growth—was a Technical Group Discussion held for one hour each week. It consisted of three 20-minute sessions on topics often decided immediately before the discussion or in the course of it.

A first short session was often devoted to analysing the dossier of a complex candidate whose performance had revealed traits not suspected from a first perusal of the paper screening. The dossier was slowly read out: the psychiatrist might comment on the projective material or health history: the psychologist on the intelligence test scores or on the educational and vocational record: the Sjt-Testers who had not dealt with this candidate might give their personal reactions. The attempt was made to find which pointers to behaviour and personality had been overlooked.

Incidentally, one training device adopted was to ask each member of the psychological team to write his comments on the dossier in a characteristic colour or medium, i.e. pen or pencil: the psychiatrist wrote his in green. In this way, the work of the Sjt-Testers could be readily identified, and each Sjt-Tester was in a position to compare the psychiatrist's subsequent interpretation with his own and to learn therefrom.

A second session might be devoted to a short seminar by the psychiatrist on a topic raised by the work: on some aspect of psychological medicine or psychodynamics: on healthy and neurotic reactions to stress: on the significance of psychosomatic complaints mentioned in the medical questionnaire: on current concepts of typology, etc. The psychologist might give a seminar in his own field: a military member of the Board might be asked to discuss the purely military aspects of the officer's role.

There was usually a 20-minute session devoted to a particular Board test or psychological procedure: its interpretation, administration, recording or improvement. Much experimentation was carried out in the presentation of Personality Pointers, Background Summaries and work-sheets: in the improvement of Interest Questionnaires, the creation of new projective questions, etc.

The team functioned to some extent as a collective in that no changes in psychological procedure inside the department were made until they had been collectively discussed, amended and approved. Co-operation and interchange of opinion with the rest of the Board were encouraged: in the hope that the psychological and job-analysis viewpoints might fertilise each other.

SELECTION PROCEDURES CANNOT FUNCTION EFFICIENTLY ON PSYCHOLOGICAL DIRECTIVES ALONE

In so far as selection is a *scientific* evaluation of abilities and personality in relation to a job, it is a psychological procedure. In so far as it considers likely physical health and mental stability on a higher level of function and responsibility, it requires medical help. In so far as it selects for a specific field and level, it needs experts in the job and the job-analysis.

To the author, it does not seem likely that a selection board can ever continue to function efficiently and maintain optimum standards on psychological directives alone: some form of continuously available psychological help on the spot seems indispensable. Certainly so, if the psychological techniques which are still tentative—both in principle and in practice—are to be further developed: and if suitable techniques are to be developed for each new special field.

Such experience as one has had of Boards that have lacked immediately available psychological help for some time is that they take a characteristic course and reveal characteristic signs. A short phase of technical insecurity seems to be followed by a phase of relative over-confidence which objective results increasingly fail to justify.

Common tendencies seem to be:—

a over-simplification of the issues and a relapse into the impressionism of "halo" and "horn" judgements:

b the re-assertion of the authority of rank as against the authority of relevant knowledge and function: and, as a consequence, the habit of mutual agreement rather than a co-operative solving of the problem:

c with (b) there may come a return of the training atmosphere as opposed to the selection atmosphere (this would be less likely in non-military fields):

d a tendency to overestimate the trainability of candidates with borderline intelligence or education but strong physical drive; and to underestimate it in complex candidates, of superior intelligence or education, whose social personality is relatively undeveloped. The function of the medical psychologist to estimate present maturity and to make a prognosis of future maturation and development is not one that can be delegated:

e the work becomes routine, uninteresting and deteriorates.

CHAPTER XX

THE VALIDATION OF BOARDS, OBSERVERS AND SELECTION PROCEDURES

By Major Gavin Reeve, M.Sc.

WHAT IS VALIDATION?

Validation is proof—proof that your selection procedure really does measure what you intend it to measure. It is also in itself a form of measurement. It measures the accuracy with which your selection procedure measures what you intend it to measure. But, before going further into the validation of WOSB, we must consider what is meant by the reliability of a measurement.

THE RELIABILITY OF A TEST

Suppose that you wanted to measure the length of an unspent match as accurately as your eyesight permitted and by means of an ordinary graduated rule.

Placing the rule against the match you might judge the length to be, say, 4.84 cms. If someone cast doubt on your measurement you might repeat it; and you might then judge that, on the first occasion, you had been mistaken in supposing the length to be just short of halfway between 4.8 cms. and 4.9 cms. and that it was, in fact, exactly halfway between these two lengths, viz. 4.85 cms., as nearly as your eye could see. If something like this occurred it would be said that your measurement of the length of the match was not perfectly reliable.

But how unreliable is it? To find this out you would have to make a small psychological experiment. You might take, say, 25 matches and measure their lengths and then having got a friend to jumble up the matches, you could measure the length of each a second time.

A colleague of the writer has carried out this experiment and his results are recorded in the diagram below.

It will be seen that 6 of the matches were judged to be 4.80 cms. long the first time they were measured, and judged to be 4.80 cms. the second time they were measured. One was judged to be 4.89 cms. the first time and 4.88 cms. the second time. One was judged to be 4.82 cms. the first time and 4.85 cms. the second time, and so on.

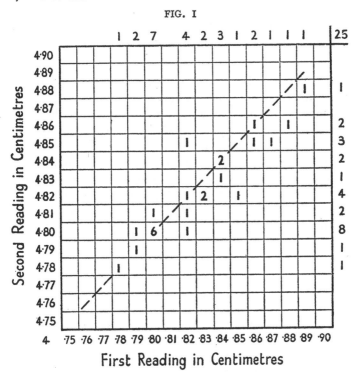

FIG. I

First Reading in Centimetres

Altogether, only 12 of the 25 matches were judged to be the same length on both the first and the second readings. These are the 1, 1, 6, 1, 2, and 1 matches which lie on the bottom left to top right diagonal of the diagram (along the dotted line). Two results emerge: one is that it is probable that the matches are, in fact, not all of exactly the same length, and the other is that the measuring of the lengths of the matches is not perfectly reliable, for had it been perfectly reliable, all the readings would lie on the bottom left to top right diagonal of the diagram (assuming no systematic or constant error which would shift the line of agreement on the paper).

Any standard textbook of statistics shows how to calculate the product-moment correlation coefficient (r) which is a measure of the closeness with which the readings are clustered about this diagonal. If all the readings lie on this diagonal, r is 1, indicating perfect correlation (in this case it would be perfect reliability of measurement). If the readings are scattered randomly over the whole diagram i.e. if there is no tendency for the first and second readings to agree r is o.

In the present case the correlation is given by

$$r = .92$$

showing a considerable extent of agreement between first and second readings, yet not perfect agreement.

We may note in passing that the average of the 25 first readings is 4.825 cms. and that the average of the 25 second readings is 4.821 cms. so that the difference in standard is practically negligible. This, however, is not relevant to the reliability of the measuring as defined above, and is a matter that would require separate treatment in any systematic investigation. We ignore the matter here as what we have presented is merely an illustrative example.

VALIDATION FORMALLY EQUIVALENT TO A MEASUREMENT OF RELIABILITY

Validation, as usually carried out, is formally identical with a measurement of reliability. If we had as our second readings a set of true and exact gradings of the officer-quality of our candidates we could use the WOSB gradings of the same candidates as our first set of readings, and the correlation coefficient, r, between the two sets of readings would be our measurement of the validity of the WOSB for the criterion we had chosen, viz., the second set of readings. The problem of validating WOSB therefore resolves itself into how and where we can find a set of gradings of the candidates which, if not perfect, is accurate enough to serve as a criterion.

THE CHOICE OF A CRITERION

What do we select people for? Primarily for success on the job. Secondarily for success in the training course, for it is useless to select candidates, however suitable they might be for the job, if the training school is to reject them either during the course or as a result of the examination at the end of it. Clearly, if all is organized to perfection, those responsible at all three stages—the selection, training and user stages—will agree as to what is required in an officer. If, in addition to this agreement, the assessors at all three stages were able to grade the candidates with perfect reliability (as defined above), we should find a perfect correlation ($r = 1$) between each pair of gradings, i.e. between gradings at the selection stage and at the training stage, between gradings at the selection stage and at the user stage, and between gradings at the training stage and at the user stage.

The proviso as to the assessors being able to grade with perfect reliability is an important one as, in general, the reliability of any set of gradings sets an upper limit to the possible validity for it of any other set of gradings. This must be borne in mind when the relative merits of various criteria are considered.

THE USER STAGE AS A CRITERION

When, for instance, it is said that selection is primarily for success on the job and only secondarily for success in training, it must be remembered that if the gradings made by the assessors at the user stage are insufficiently reliable, we can learn very little from them as to the value of our selection procedure and very little as to the value of the gradings made at the training stage. In addition to this, the charges of fallibility so widely and, to a large extent so justly, preferred against human judgement may lie against assessors at the user stage as against those at any other stage. In short, the efficiency of the Army in the field is not identical with the success of individual officers in the Army because the success in the Army of individual officers depends on the gradings of their seniors whose judgement in such matters, like all human judgement, is more or less fallible.

Apart from such considerations, there are practical difficulties in employing as a criterion gradings made at the user stage. The number of different military units is so large that it is difficult to draw a sample of candidates of manageable size that has more than a very few members whose efficiency is assessed by the same Commanding Officer; and different Commanding Officers are liable to have different standards which would result in differences corresponding to the difference between the two averages 4.825 cms. and 4.821 cms. in our example of the matches. Also, the military units are so scattered that it is difficult for technical staff to visit them to give Commanding Officers the technical advice which is necessary if gradings of adequate reliability are to be achieved. In addition to this, the posting of candidates and of assessing officers from one unit to another introduces wide variation into the times during which an assessing officer has known the various candidates he is required to assess.

We do hope, however, to make some use of the gradings from training courses which some serving officers attend from time to time, as a field criterion both for WOSB and for OCTU gradings.

THE TRAINING STAGE AS A CRITERION

The training stage as a criterion is free from many of the difficulties of the user stage. The number of OCTUs is not large and most of them are situated in the United Kingdom where they are accessible to technical staff. The candidates, of course, remain at the OCTUs for a specified time and changes of assessing staff are not unduly frequent. The OCTUs have a continuity of training policy which is far more stable than the circumstances of many units serving in the field and, with it, has become associated a continuity of policy of assessment. On the other hand the OCTUs, although nearer to the user stage than are the WOSBs, are still one degree removed from it, so that their gradings must contain an element of prophecy from which gradings at the user stage are free.

WHAT DO WE EXPECT FROM OCTU GRADINGS AS A CRITERION?

The essential task of a WOSB is to distinguish between those candidates who will, after success in the training course, make useful officers and those who would either fail the training course or, should they somehow pass it, would still not make useful officers. That is, a WOSB's essential task is to decide rightly which candidates it should accept and which it should reject. The gradings it allots to the successful candidates are not communicated to the OCTUs and are not entered in the candidate's documents, so that they have little or no administrative consequence. They serve a useful purpose in promoting clarity and precision of thought in the assessing officers at WOSBs; but, from the point of view of validation, their principal function is as a means of measuring the skill with which Boards and individuals on Boards can discriminate between candidates of different calibre. It is assumed, though it cannot be proved, that a Board or an individual who can distinguish well between candidates who will achieve a high OCTU grading and candidates who will achieve a low one will also be good at distinguishing between candidates who will succeed at OCTU and in the field and candidates who will fail at either of these two stages. This assumption must remain unproved, or at best only partially proved, because although we learn in due course of candidates whom the WOSBs mistakenly accept, we can rarely, if ever, have direct knowledge of those whom they mistakenly reject. A low RTU rate at the OCTUs could generally be obtained by creaming off only the best of the candidates at WOSBs, but this would involve the rejection of a great many candidates who would have made successful officers which is, in general, undesirable.

It will be seen therefore, that in using OCTU gradings as a criterion we are measuring the skill of our selection units in distinguishing between the merits of accepted candidates as a means of estimating their relative capacity to distinguish between those who should be accepted and those who should be rejected. It is not to be supposed that the judgement of the assessing officers at OCTUs is infallible, nor that in every case of disagreement the OCTUs are right and the WOSBs are wrong. It is simply that two independent opinions, when they agree, can be accepted with greater assurance than one unsupported opinion. Cross comparisons frequently clarify the situation further. For instance, if all the WOSBs except one agree with the OCTUs in a certain respect it is reasonable to assume provisionally that the fault lies in the minority party and investigation of its psychological procedure may add confirmation to the diagnosis. Similarly if all the OCTUs except one agree with the WOSBs a psychological fault may be revealed at that OCTU. If, when these faults are rectified, the unit concerned yields figures that fall into line with the others, further confirmation is added. In general, the degree of confidence we are entitled to feel in our choice and use of our criterion must depend upon the extent to which such detailed observations fall into place to make up a consistent picture.

THE EFFECT OF SELECTION ON THE MEASURED VALIDITY

It was mentioned above that, although we know from the failures at OCTU how many candidates were mistakenly accepted by WOSBs, we cannot in general have any direct knowledge of how many were mistakenly rejected. This inevitable lack of information about the rejected WOSB candidates has a marked effect upon our measurement of the validity of WOSB and, if this effect is not borne in mind, we may seriously under-estimate the efficiency of our selection procedure.

In our example of the matches, all twenty-five matches that were measured the first time were available for measurement the second time. In the case of WOSB, out of every 100 candidates tested only about 33 are accepted. It follows that when we wish to compare the first and second measurements of our candidates—their WOSB and OCTU gradings—we are confined to approximately one-third of our original population. If in the case of our matches we strike out the 16 shortest matches as judged by the first measurement, regarding these as candidates rejected by WOSB, and calculate the correlation for the remaining 9 matches (accepted by WOSB and therefore sent to OCTU), we obtain a validity given by

$$r = .83$$

And yet the larger figure (.92) is the fairer measure of the closeness of the relation between the two sets of measurements.

Methods are available of estimating from the figures of the smaller population what is the likely correlation between the measurements for the whole population; but these methods can be employed only when certain conditions obtain and it frequently happens that they do not do so.

Evidence now available shows that these conditions are not, in general, fulfilled by the WOSB and OCTU gradings, so that although future changes in psychological and statistical procedure might make available to us figures that do satisfy the conditions, we are at present confined to the use of validities on the selected group of candidates (those accepted by WOSBs).

This restriction prevents us from using our correlations (except within very wide limits) to compare the efficiency of WOSB with that of any other working system of selection that might be proposed, and which had a very different rejection rate; but it does not prevent us from comparing the efficiency of one WOSB or of one assessor at a WOSB with that of another, or with its own efficiency at a different time or with candidates of a different type, and for practical purposes these are the comparisons we need to make. They direct attention to more and to less efficient elements in our selection machinery on which psychological attention can then be concentrated. In this way we are enabled to reinforce the more efficient elements, rectify the less efficient, and so progressively improve the efficiency of selection.

AN INSTANCE OF VALIDATION

In the left-hand diagram below we have plotted the relation between the WOSB and OCTU gradings of 33 candidates who were successful at the OCTU. In the right-hand diagram we have plotted the relation between the OCTU gradings of these same candidates and the gradings proposed for them at the WOSB by a particular member of the assessing officers who, as is to be expected, differs from the Board itself to some extent in the gradings he considered appropriate to some of the candidates.

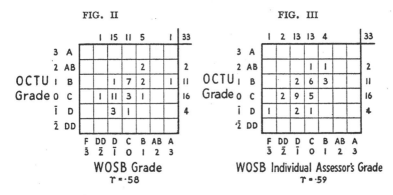

The grades, unlike the measurements of the lengths of the matches, must have numerical values arbitrarily assigned to them, and we have assigned the simplest possible values (-3 to $+3$ for WOSB grades and -2 to $+3$ for OCTU grades. The zeros are placed at the centres of the grades C purely for arithmetical convenience. A number of problems arise in connection with choice of these numerical scales, but it is not possible to discuss them here. Another matter that must be noted without detailed explanation is that, in this sample of candidates, D is the modal or most frequently occurring WOSB grade (15 candidates were so graded in the left-hand diagram), whereas C is the modal OCTU grade (16 of the candidates being so graded). This has to do with a difference of standard such as we spoke of in the example of the matches and with a difference between the grading procedure at the WOSBs and the OCTUs. The correlations (.58 and .59) are unaffected by this. It is not, of course, surprising that the two correlations should be so nearly the same, because the individual assessor has contributed his opinion towards the official grading of the Board.

There are, however, differences in the cases of a number of individual candidates. This can be seen more clearly by studying the above two diagrams in conjunction with that given below which shows the relation between the Board's gradings and those given by the individual member.

FIG. IV

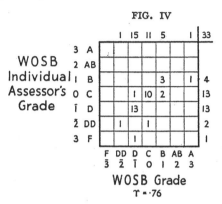

WOSB Individual Assessor's Grade

WOSB Grade

T = ·76

Fig. II shows that one candidate was considered by the Board to be outstandingly good and accordingly graded A. It shows also that the OCTU considered him good but not outstandingly so, as they graded him B which is a lower grade than they allotted to two other members of the sample.

Fig. IV shows that the individual assessor did not agree that he was better than all the others, for he graded him B (the highest grading he used for any member of the sample) but equal to three others. Thus, in the case of this candidate, the OCTU tends to agree with the individual assessor rather than with the Board. It remains to be seen whether the candidate's subsequent career in the Army will tend to support one view rather than the other.

On the other hand, Fig. IV shows that the individual assessor recommended the rejection of one candidate by grading him F, although the Board decided to accept him and graded him D. Fig. III shows that this candidate passed out of OCTU with the grade of D. In this case, then, the OCTU has tended to confirm the opinion of the Board rather than that of the individual assessor; and again, the candidate's subsequent career in the Army may tend to support one view or the other.

These validities (.58 and .59) have been obtained on a group of candidates that has been reduced by selection to about one-third of its original size; but it will be seen that they are, nevertheless, smaller than the value .83 obtained as the reliability of the measurements of the lengths of matches on a similarly reduced group. This is, perhaps, not surprising in view of the far greater complexity and difficulty of assessing qualities of human character for which no objectively graded steel or wooden rule is available.

THE CONTRIBUTION OF A PARTICULAR PSYCHIATRIST TO THE VALIDITY OF A WOSB

As one further example of validation, we present some results from an investigation into the contribution to selection of interviews by a particular psychiatrist.

The sample studied consists of 119 candidates. The validity of the Board's final grading on the whole sample of 119 is given by
$$r = .14$$

Such a low value as this might well be due to the chances of sampling, so that so far we have little or no evidence that any relation at all subsists between the WOSB and OCTU gradings for candidates other than those in the sample. However, on dividing the 119 candidates into the 57 interviewed by the psychiatrist we are studying and the 62 not interviewed by him, we find that the validity of the Board is .43 for the 57 and − .14 for the 62. Comparable differences appear between the Team Leaders' validities and between the PSOs' validities for the two groups of candidates. The results may be tabulated as follows:—

FIG. V

	Validity of Gradings given by:—			
	PSO	Team Leader	The Board	The Psychiatrist being studied
For the 57 Candidates Interviewed by the Psychiatrist being studied	·43	·35	·43	·38
For the 62 Candidates not Interviewed by the Psychiatrist being Studied	−.07	−.11	−.14	—

The difference between the two members of each of these 3 pairs of validities is larger than is likely to have arisen as a result of the chances of sampling.

Of the 62 candidates, 41 were interviewed by another psychiatrist, 12 by a psychologist and 9 by neither a psychiatrist nor a psychologist.

It is not possible to deal here with a number of considerations (such as how the candidates were allotted for interview by this particular psychiatrist) which must be borne in mind if we are to assure ourselves as far as possible that the differences between the validities are not due to some extraneous cause or causes. We can only record that after careful consideration it is concluded that in all probability the figures are a genuine reflection of an effect of this psychiatrist's work in raising the selective efficiency of the Board in the terms in which we have chosen to measure it from effectively zero to an appreciable and, as many will think, a satisfactory value in view of the highly selected nature of the group of candidates.

It seems unlikely that, even when it is working at zero, validity (as we measure it) the WOSB is exerting no selective influence at all. On the other hand, it seems reasonable to suppose that when a WOSB's gradings of its successful candidates are largely confirmed by the opinion of the assessors at OCTUs, then its judgement as to whom to accept and whom to reject is the more to be trusted.

A USE OF AVERAGES

In our example of the matches the averages for the first and for the second groups of measurements were very little different, but in our selection data the average OCTU grading is within C and the average WOSB grading is within D. It has been pointed out that the validities are independent of the standards set by the assessors as shown by these averages; nevertheless the averages can themselves yield information of practical use.

It was found that, over a period of many months, one of the WOSBs was consistently rejecting a somewhat larger percentage of candidates than was each of the others, so that the question arose as to whether this WOSB was more exacting than the others or whether it was merely receiving candidates whose quality was, on the average, relatively poor. A random sample of 300 candidates (successful at OCTUs and graded A to DD at WOSBs) was available such that 10 had proceeded from each of 6 WOSBs to each of 5 OCTUs. The mean WOSB grading and the mean OCTU grading of the 50 candidates from each WOSB was calculated and plotted as in Fig. VI.

FIG. VI

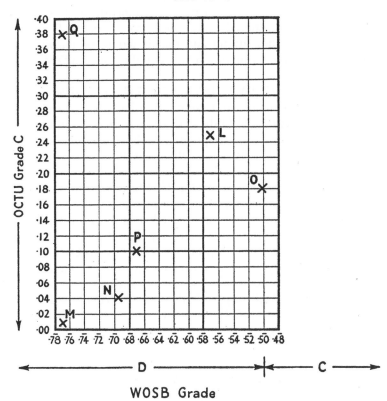

WOSB Grade

The WOSBs are named L, M, N, O, P and Q. Q is the WOSB which had shown a rather higher rejection rate than the others, from which, it will be seen, it tends to stand apart. Together with WOSB M it gives the lowest average of WOSB gradings; yet, so far from its candidates achieving low OCTU gradings, they achieve, on the average, higher OCTU gradings than the candidates from any of the other WOSBs. The investigation is subject to certain limitations into which we cannot enter here, and it required to be supplemented by a more detailed study of the gradings of larger numbers of candidates, but the general result is to suggest that WOSB Q is more exacting in its requirements of candidates than are the 5 other WOSBs and that there is no need to suppose that it has received, on the average, candidates of poorer quality.

In this way differences of standard between WOSBs can be detected and can then be rectified. It is important that, as far as possible, candidates should have the same chance of passing whichever WOSB they attend and that it should be known that every effort is made to maintain this equality of standards.

A USE OF RTU RATES (FAILURE RATES) AT OCTUS.

It has been pointed out that information about candidates mistakenly accepted by WOSBs is of only limited value because it cannot, in general, be supplemented by information about candidates mistakenly rejected by them. Nevertheless, there are circumstances in which practical use can be made of it.

At one time it was customary for WOSBs to accept candidates whom they considered satisfactory except that they were unduly immature. Such candidates were ungraded except for the pseudo-grading "148" which indicated that they should receive a special course of training in leadership before being sent to OCTU.

It was necessary for administrative reasons to cancel this special course of training and thereafter candidates who would have been graded "148" by WOSBs were graded instead "DY" and sent forward to OCTUs without any special training. A comparison thus became possible between the OCTU results of 192 "148s", 105 "DYs" and 400 ordinary WOSB "Ds", all of whom had emerged from the OCTUs over the same period. It was found that the distributions of the OCTU gradings of the successful candidates of the three groups did not differ significantly but that the RTU (Return to Unit) rate of the "DYs" was approximately double that of the "148s" and that of the "Ds", the differences being statistically significant. Such figures direct attention to psychological problems requiring solution and enable administrative action to be taken.

The inclusion in calculations of candidates who were unsuccessful at OCTUs is restricted by the time-lag which results from numerous candidates being relegated to later courses at the OCTUs if they are tending to fall behind their colleagues.

In conclusion, however, we present the RTU rates amongst candidates of various WOSB grades taken over a very extensive period. The number of RTUs are those who were actually returned to their units (for reasons other than medical or compassionate) during the period covered by the pass-out dates of the successful candidates.

FIG. VII

WOSB Final Grade	RTUs	Passes	Totals	% RTU Rate
A	0	7	7	0.0%
AB	0	3	3	0.0%
B	5	171	176	2.8%
C	32	868	900	3.6%
D	158	1570	1728	9.1%
DD	4	40	44	9.1%
"148"	121	906	1027	11.8%

It is clear that candidates of high WOSB grade tend to have a lower RTU rate at OCTU than do candidates of low WOSB grade. The results also confirm, what we have other reasons to suppose, namely, that WOSB distinguishes less sharply between candidates of low WOSB grade than between candidates of higher WOSB grade. If WOSB is to provide the administration with a means of controlling the RTU rate in the light of the number of trained officers required and the training accommodation available at OCTUs, it will need to develop its discrimination between candidates of low WOSB grade.

STANDARDS AND SOME OTHER PROBLEMS

So far, we have given examples of the validation (by means of correlation coefficients) of boards and of individual members of boards and we have shown a simple use of percentage failure-rates at WOSBs and at OCTUs. We have also shown how use can be made of a comparison between the standards at different WOSBs as shown by the averages of the gradings they allot; but we have not considered the question of defining the standards. A working definition is clearly necessary and has been employed, but the problem of finding the best definition has proved more complex than was first expected.

We may illustrate the problem—or some aspects of it—by referring again to our example of the matches. It will be seen that amongst the first measurements of the 25 matches the measurement that occurred most frequently (7 times) is not in the middle of the scale but towards its lower end (actually at 4.80 cms.), and that a similar effect occurs amongst the second measurements of which the greatest number (8) occur again towards the lower end (at 4.80 cms.). Thus the distribution of

I

the measurements is not symmetrical about their average, but is skewed to one side. If matches were the object of our study we should first verify, on a larger sample, that this skewed form of distribution really was typical of the matches in general and then look for the cause of it, perhaps in the machinery with which the match sticks were cut into lengths, or in the viscosity of the igniting material into which they were dipped, or in some other part of their manufacture. And we might find that matches manufactured under different conditions gave different forms of distribution. In the same way we are beginning to find that the gradings of candidates of different types and the gradings of candidates made under different conditions give different forms of distribution; and this serves to increase our knowledge of the candidates and of the psychological processes of grading them. It is also relevant to the definition of standards. Better definition of standards will lead to greater precision of grading both at WOSBs and at OCTUs and this, in turn, will give us more sensitive tests of differences between good and bad selection.

The seventeen profile-items mentioned in Chapter XVIII, provide an alternative means of classifying the candidates, and the results can be compared with a number of somewhat similar profile assessments of the same candidates made at OCTU.

The full use that can be made of the profile-items will not be known until a very extensive study of them has been made; but we have employed them to validate WOSBs for OCTU final gradings on candidates graded "148" at WOSBs.

"148" is not a grading in the sense that A to DD are gradings. "148" means simply that a candidate is expected to pass successfully out of OCTU provided his OCTU training is preceded by a special course of training elsewhere to remedy to some extent the effects of his immaturity. It gives no indication of whether the candidate is expected to do well or less well at OCTU, so that the grading cannot be included in the grading scale A to DD.

The way out of the difficulty is to construct for each "148" candidate an artificial WOSB grading consisting of the sum of his gradings on the seventeen profile-items—not just the simple sum, but a weighted sum, say 3 times his score on Quality of Personal Relations plus twice his score on Leadership Experience, and so on—mixing them up in set proportions like a bottle of medicine. The proportions are calculated beforehand, from the profile-gradings of a very large sample of candidates, as being those proportions that give the highest possible correlation with the OCTU gradings. In the case of candidates with WOSB gradings A to DD, this statistical integration provides an interesting comparison with the corresponding integration of the same material that takes place in the minds of the assessors in so far as they depend on the profile-gradings in forming their final grading of the candidates. This method is not infrequently used to combine the scores on a number of educational and psychological tests into a single comprehensive score, but more work requires to be done on it before it can make a contribution to practical selection at WOSB. It has, however, yielded some statistically significant results which are suggestive for research purposes.

Limitation of space prevents us from describing a number of other investigations which have given us useful knowledge of the detailed functioning of WOSB. For instance, it has been found that, in general, WOSBs and OCTUs agree more closely (give a significantly higher correlation) as regards the merits of candidates from some types of schools than of those from others. This is not a question of candidates from some types of schools being of better quality than those from other types of schools, but of the skill with which assessors distinguish the better from the less good candidates within each separate type of school. Clearly, psychiatrists and psychologists must discover the means of raising the efficiency of WOSB and/or OCTU to its maximum on all types of candidates.

So far we have not measured the contribution of separate parts of the testing procedure towards the validity of the whole, but the introduction of the GABI rank-rating system at intermediate stages should help us to do this. This should be a big step forward.

I*

PART 3: TRENDS AND IMPLICATIONS

CHAPTER XXI

LEADERSHIP TESTING IN OTHER THAN MILITARY FIELDS

G AND S FACTORS IN LEADERSHIP

The possible existence of g and s factors in leadership is considered in Chapters IV and V. On the one hand there seem to be factors that contribute to leadership in any field (they determine group-cohesiveness and the intelligence and educational components of functional level): on the other hand there seem to be factors whose contribution is specific to a particular field (they determine the remaining components of functional level i.e. special aptitudes and special attitudes or identifications with a special field). The s factors contribute to a man's total effective leadership only when he is working in that special field. Both g and s factors condition stability on any level.

Among the g factors, group-cohesiveness stands out: among the s factors, emotional identification with the particular field seems important.

WOSB TECHNIQUES FOR ESTIMATING G FACTORS ARE TRANSFERABLE TO OTHER FIELDS

This book deals with the g factors as investigated in WOSB: s factors—specific to the military field—are only incidentally mentioned. The thesis is that these g factors exist and that their investigation will be of value in selection for leadership in any field: in industry, the civil and military services, the professions, teaching, medicine, nursing, the social and other sciences, the guidance of entrants to universities and of graduates to fields of activity, etc. In some of these fields, techniques derivative from WOSB have already been initiated.

S FACTORS MUST BE WORKED OUT FOR EACH INDIVIDUAL FIELD

The s factors will have to be worked out for each individual field.

Much more might be known about the relationship between special aptitudes and specific emotional attitudes. One would like to know, for instance, whether high ratings in a spatial factor or in kinaesthetic ability and muscular co-ordination might predispose to a stronger identification with material things or with their manipulation in physical skills. Whether verbal facility is likely to increase the emotional identification with people and with social interests generally: or whether it can be increased by such an identification. Whether high intelligence—in the absence of marked kinaesthetic or verbal aptitudes or interests—will tend to orient the individual towards ideas and abstract thinking.

THE RELATIONSHIP BETWEEN SPECIAL APTITUDES AND SPECIAL ATTITUDES

Much work remains to be done here by psychologists, medical psychologists and job-analysts in team. One's own experience in helping to direct several thousand potential officers to a variety of technical and non-technical Arms leaves one with these clinical impressions:—

a in selection on leadership level, aptitudes matter less and attitudes matter more than is generally thought:

b special aptitudes (i.e. potential skills as distinct from trained acquired skills) may not vary as widely as is commonly thought; and the effects of training and interest may be greater:

c most major fields of activity offer scope for a wide range of special aptitudes i.e. in medicine, one may be physician, surgeon, psychotherapist, administrator, laboratory-worker, statistician, teacher, etc.:

d a strong emotional identification with a special field— even if compensatory for a real or apparent lack of special aptitude—can powerfully influence trainability and ultimate capacity in that field: its effect is more often under-estimated than over-estimated.

TWO TYPES OF PROJECTIVE TECHNIQUE TO REVEAL ATTITUDES

One cannot work on selection teams without realising the importance of emotional attitudes to the job and to interests allied with it. The projective techniques, integral to WOSB, aim at revealing emotional attitudes both to the group and to the job. Because of that, they are—one is tempted to repeat—the germinating point of leadership-testing techniques.

Projective sessions of these two kinds can be invaluable:—

a A Human Problems Session aimed at projecting for the most part the individual's *attitude to the group and the group-purpose*, i.e. his group-cohesiveness.

b A vocational session aimed to project his *attitude to the job* and interests allied with it: and which may combine many elements from the Apparatus Session with the projective techniques of the Human Problems Session. It might include individual talks of the type: "What I like most (and/or least) about engineering, teaching, etc., etc.": "What I should do to improve engineering, teaching, etc., etc.": also quizzes, criticisms and counter-criticisms by the group generally.

BOARD PROCEDURES FOR NON-MILITARY FIELDS

The following general points occur to one:—

a The 3-phase board is by far the simplest, easiest and most productive.

b One envisages if possible a board in which every member observes every test: except for the paper screening.

c In the paper-screening, there is scope for the development and more systematic use of Interest Questionnaires to cover the job and interests fringing on it.

d The physical and outdoor situations used in WOSB—however interesting and valuable—might have been dispensed with, even in the military field. In other fields, the emphasis should pass to projective and planning sessions which, in conjunction with tests of general and special aptitude and linked interviews, should provide a clear picture of the candidate's suitability for further training for leadership responsibility.

e A suggested pattern of testing is given below:—

Phase 1. A Basic Series containing:

1 An unorganised and undirected Group Discussion of a general nature lasting at least an hour.

2 A project in 2 stages:

> *a* a planning stage in which the candidate is given a dossier of the details and prepares his written plan:
>
> *b* a committee or leaderless group stage in which candidates meet to deal with the problem.

Phase 2. To contain in addition to the interviews:

> 1 A Group Discussion of a directed nature whose topic is related to the job or interests fringing on it.
>
> 2 A Vocational or Interests Session as described above.

Phase 3. This might use a Human Problems Session to allow a last projection of the social personality of the candidate. The situation is not a simple leaderless group. One sees him, *not* in the general context of the group, but spot-lighted against it: interacting for part of the time with one other member of the group (i.e. the Stooge) in a specific man-management role: and for part of the time with the group as a whole.

f Much simpler procedures can of course be used if their tested validity justifies them for their particular purpose.

SELECTING FOR FOREMAN OR NCO LEVEL

The Army screened and selected its troops on 2 levels (1) on aptitude level to distribute them to the appropriate Arm and job, i.e. driver, signaller, clerk, infanteer, etc.: (2) on officer level. In the first screening, those whose potential functional level seemed to justify it, were ear-marked for WOSB: others were noted as potential NCOs.

There seems every reason why one should—in industry and in the military services—grade the levels intermediate between officership and the lowest rank. This might be done at either or both of the screenings mentioned above. It seems a pity that those rejected by selection boards should undergo so intensive an investigation without grading, advice or direction towards their appropriate functional level. Such a grading would be useful both to the candidate and the community: if subsequently followed up, it would act both as a check on selection board procedure and as a safeguard for the candidate.

One's own estimate of the average range of functional level on NCO or foreman level is an OIR of about 3 to 5 (roughly from the 65th to the 85th percentile of the population on intelligence score) and an Educational Standard of about 5 (school up to the age of 15).

So far as group-cohesiveness is concerned, one may on this level have to tolerate—without encouraging—a larger element of the dominant type of leadership (dependent on physical qualities or the arbitrary exercise of vested authority by word of command) than one would on officer level. But if this can be eliminated by better selection, training and morale, it will be an important step forward in the evolution of leadership.

SELECTING WOMEN FOR LEADERSHIP

WOSB techniques—based on the same general principles but with modifications in detail—were used to select ATS officers. Specific differences in the traits and roles to be investigated in tests and psychological profile have still to be more precisely considered and defined.

One sees no reason why mixed Boards should not select mixed candidates. Some of the special temptations that all-women boards may succumb to, are:—

   a to follow masculine models too closely: especially in the maintenance of a training atmosphere of firm discipline where the need is for a selection atmosphere that relaxes and de-tenses the candidate:

   b a difficulty—that should be obvious enough—in being objective about candidates who happen to be attractive to men.

   c a relative lack of objectivity about differences in socio-economic status, accent, etc.

Intuition is a splendid and necessary thing in the judgement process, if harnessed to a discipline of self-analysis and objectivity. The sin is *not* in having personal prejudices but in failing to allow for them.

CHAPTER XXII

PARTICIPATION IN COLLECTIVE LEADERSHIP AS A TRUE SOCIAL INCENTIVE

In *The Hero in History* (page 163), Sidney Hook makes the following comments (the italics are mine):—

"*It is the task of a democratic society to break down the invidious distinctions reflected in current linguistic usage between the hero and the masses or the average man.* This can be accomplished in part by reinterpreting the meaning of the word "hero", *and by recognising that* "*heroes*" *can be made by fitting social opportunities more skilfully to specific talents.* What we call "the average man" is not a biological but a social phenomenon. Human capacities are much more diversified than our social arrangements take note of.

"When we restrict social opportunities, so that only a few types of excellence are recognised, in respect to them the great mass of individuals, despite their differences, will appear as the dull, grey average. If however we extend social opportunities so that each person's specific talents have a stimulus to development and expression, we increase the range of possibility of distinctively significant work. *From this point of view, a hero is any individual who does his work well and makes a unique contribution to the public good.* It is sheer prejudice to believe that the grandeur and nobility associated with the heroic life can be found only in careers that reck little of human blood and suffering. Daily toil on any level has its own occasions of struggle, victory and quiet death. *A democracy should contrive its affairs, not to give one or a few the chance to reach heroic stature, but rather to take as a regulative ideal the slogan* "*every man a hero*".

"*We call this a 'regulative ideal' because it would be Utopian to imagine that it could ever be literally embodied. As a regulative ideal it gives direction to policies that enable society to make the best of whatever powers are available to men.*

". . . *A democracy should encourage the belief that all are called and all may be chosen.* All may be chosen because a wisely contrived society will take as a point of departure the rich possibilities that Nature herself gives through the spontaneous variations in the powers and capacities of men. These variations are the source and promise of new shoots of personality and value. *The belief that all may be chosen, acted upon in a co-operating environment, may inspire the added increment of effort that often transforms promise into achievement."*

"EVERY MAN A LEADER" AS A TRUE INCENTIVE

May I suggest that if we substitute for "hero" the word "leader", as in this book defined, we have a real and comprehensive incentive—perhaps the only truly democratic one—one that may liberate the "atomic energy" of the human spirit. A true incentive, as distinct from those so-called "negative incentives"—fear of the sack, fear that those one cherishes will become destitute—which I prefer to term "compulsions".

For, while incentives should induce a willing contribution and a happy spontaneous use of one's faculties, compulsions can only drive the unwilling spirit. They are extravagant in human energy because they compel one to use energy not only to do the job but also to drive oneself *to* the job.

COMMENSURATE GROUP-EFFECTIVENESS AS A SIGN OF SOCIAL HEALTH

To quote from Chapter IV in this book:—

"What seems to emerge is that every man should be capable of some degree of leadership—influencing others towards a satisfying participation in collective effort; and being sensitive to the influence of others—on his own level and in his own field of activity: and one might regard it as a basic sign of mental and social health that he show some degree of effective, happy and spontaneous leadership on that level. In that sense every man should be a leader.

" . . . Leadership then may be regarded as the expression of a man's adequately realised group-effectiveness on his own natural level: neurosis, as the indication and result of an inadequately realised group-effectiveness; of some impediment (be it external, internal or both) in the realisation of his potential group-effectiveness, natural leadership and capacity for zestful living."

LEADERSHIP AS A COLLECTIVE FUNCTION

To quote again from Chapter XII:—

"Leadership is a collective function: collective in the sense that it is the integrated synergised expression of a group's efforts: it can only arise in relation to a group problem or purpose; it is not the sum of individual dominances and contributions, it is their relationship."

"In so far as a man contributes to the collective leadership function . . . he will realise that the ultimate authority and true sanction for leadership, at every point where it is exercised, resides—not in the individual, however dominant, strong or efficient he may be—but in the 'total situation' and in the demands of that situation, i.e. the Law of the Total Situation. It is the situation that creates the imperative, not the individual. To the extent that the individual is aware of that imperative, is able to make others aware of it, is able to make them willing to serve it: to the extent that he is able to release collective capacities and emotional attitudes that may be related fruitfully to the solution of the group's problems: to that extent he is exercising leadership. He will realise that a two-fold link—functional *and* emotional—between the group and the LOTS is implicit in any leadership that is effective: and that it is this two-fold link· that makes leadership inevitably a collective function in which human drives and human abilities and skills are harnessed to cooperate with the environment."

COOPERATION A RESPONSE TO INCENTIVE; COMPETITION— TO COMPULSION

Because leadership is a collective function exercised to solve the problems and assure the security of the group, the co-operative attitude is more acceptable to the group than the competitive.

Those who exaggerate the influence of competition on the biological evolution of man, and underestimate the importance of cooperation (one cannot imagine man evolving unless there were a predominance of the latter) will tend to think that the best products of man are a result of the competitive spirit. Even a superficial understanding of the psychodynamics of man should reveal the fallacy of this belief: which seems to be a projection of one's own unresolved aggression.

The cooperative attitude helps both helped and helper in a binding relationship. Success in competition is more likely to arouse ill-will than good-will: if it encourages the one to the extent and risk of inflating his ego, it discourages the many:

as it increases in intensity it tends to associate itself with a cult of purposeful ruthlessness—a search for "power *over*" rather than "power *with*", to use the terms of Mary Parker Follett—which is more likely to lead to a bad conscience than a good one.

The cooperative attitude is cohesive, creative, and—because it leads to one's acceptance by the group—a source of enduring security. The competitive attitude is ultimately disruptive and destructive; it can never lead to unequivocal acceptance by the group or to any real sense of security. The likelihood is that its desire to surpass derives from the compulsions of an inner sense of inadequacy rather than from genuine incentives; and goes on to feed those compulsions by failing to gain any real acceptance from the group. No technical success or superiority can give it the warm enduring security of the group: at best these can give only the transient tingle of narcissistic self-satisfaction. It is the individualist "Führer-prinzip" of the man who leads mankind for his own benefit to their own undoing.

The so-called "socialistic competition" that culminates in Stakhanovism is not so much competition as a dramatisation of the force of example. By making the good example so vividly explicit, and by overemphasising the individual component in collective effort, it runs the risk—by odious comparisons and a tincture of true competition—of lowering morale more than it raises it. It is a fighting term, coined by those who feel in terms of conflict; analogous to the advocacy of the Christianity of Love by those who talk of warriors and battles in the terminology of organised Hate.

Even if the competitive attitude has survival-value for the individual, it may be the survival-value of the weed: not necessarily to be encouraged at the expense of the fruitful crop: and if the community disapproves of it, it will cease to have even that survival value. Psychodynamically, the competitive attitude and ideal seems to be a compulsion to surpass—to have power *over* people, to be successful *over* others—that derives from some inadequacy: it tends to lower the morale of the losers and to saddle the winner with guilt and ultimate lowering of morale: its total and ultimate achievements must be more disruptive and destructive than otherwise.

The cooperative attitude and ideal derives from a true incentive: the desire to participate in a collective function which extends one's faculties and so gives one a sufficient variety of

K

interest: which uses one effectively and gives one appreciation, prestige and security: in short, from the desire to be accepted as a worthy participant in a useful and necessary task. One might propose a "fifth freedom" to participate fruitfully and satisfyingly on one's own natural level and in a suitable field.

The efforts of the artist who hopes ultimately to communicate his "values" for the enrichment of others—insofar as they are necessarily solitary—still fall of course within the circle of co-operative effort. Other more personal joys—in nature, the inanimate, etc.—which are important to many, can only hope to develop sanely within the security and warmth bestowed by the group.

HOW IMPLEMENT THE INCENTIVE?

We have here defined leadership, social health and neurosis in terms of social and collective function; and have suggested that the incentive "all are called and all may be chosen" is one most likely to raise the morale and effectiveness of groups and individuals. It is likely that where a man's effectiveness lies, so will much of his interest: but the complete balancing of his interests need not be expected from his role in the working group: the increasing scope of leisure should be capable of absorbing such interests as are left over.

In so far as selection provides a democratic filter which aims to sift each man to his optimum level and to prevent his falling below his range of potential effectiveness, to that extent it will implement this incentive and make of it a reality.

What selection must not do—nor seem to do—is:—

a to skim the cream of the talent and neglect the rest:

b to fail to use to the fullest the handicapped, the neurotic, the disabled, the old, etc.; in short, to fail to use all the community:

c to fail to give special attention to the aggressive disruptives, i.e. either by special placement, training, rehabilitation, therapy, control, etc.:

d to fail to consider simultaneously and objectively the interest of both employer and employee, of group and member:

e to be used so rigidly or so infrequently as to seal the fate of individuals rather than *to open a gate—and keep on opening gates—to* opportunity and *further development.*

SKIMMING THE CREAM DISRUPTS THE COMMUNITY

If firms or organisations or services are allowed to skim the
cream of talent without reference to the rest of the community,
the requirements of the job or the psychological effect on those
it rejects, the accumulative effects of such discriminations will
have a disrupting and demoralising influence on the community.
All organisations that select must take their proper share of a
sufficiently wide cross-section of the community: if they skim the
cream to use greater talents for lesser jobs, they are defrauding
both the individual and the community.

THE WEAK LINKS CAN BECOME THE STRONGEST

Because those who feel themselves to be useful and effective
in a community will cement and bind it and those who do not
will become foci of psychic infection and low morale and disrupt
it, it is important that a community should take special care to
use to the full the handicapped, disabled, neurotic, old, etc.

If those who are physically or mentally handicapped are
rehabilitated, specially re-trained and found a stabilising role in
the group, it will have important effects both on themselves and
the group.

On themselves, it will have the effect of doubly binding them
to the group: firstly because of their very real conscious need for
additional security, secondly out of gratitude for the opportunity
to maintain self-respect. Just as a fractured collar-bone when
set is stronger than the original, so the weaker member who is
helped to a useful role will become a stronger link in the social
pattern which he both respects and needs.

On the group, it has the effect of giving them a good conscience and an enhanced sense of security. For they surely know
that health or age or act of Providence may impair any man's
usefulness. A community which scraps its weaker members is a
pretty poor group: that it gives its stronger members greater
rewards while they remain strong enough to earn them is no
redeeming feature: its morale is a brittle one, easily disrupted.
Much "ca-canny" in the response of workers may be resentment
of such an attitude. No firm or organisation or community will
be so loved as that known to use skilfully and without loss of face
or morale its weaker, less stable or older members: none will
reap so rich a reward of gratitude and loyalty.

A similar strengthening of the community will accrue from

its handling of "the bottom 10%" of the population so far as intelligence (as indicated by test scores) is concerned. They contribute too large a percentage to be rejected or carried or dealt with by any short-term eugenic or euthenic program: their capacity for mischief and disruption is sufficiently great, and it would certainly be short-sighted to allow them to become dependent, delinquent or demoralised. They will always need and appreciate "elder-brotherly" guidance and help from the abler majority of the communal family.

That their morale and effectiveness and happiness can be raised to a high degree was amply proved in the large-scale techniques devised for their disposal, training and use by the British Army in 1941-45. Quite outstanding was the reduction in illness and delinquency; the increase in work, morale and happiness; their cheering effect on the abler members of their service.

A recurrent problem in history—and a sufficiently serious one—is the war veteran, disabled or not, who has not been helped back to the fold. No pension can substitute for the feeling of being needed or useful. It was especially true of the psychiatric casualties of the 1914-18 war that too many—through lack of immediate or sufficient therapy or adequate rehabilitation—were allowed to become dependent, permanently pensionable, ineffective and disgruntled members of society: permanent foci of psychic infection and low morale.

A realisation of this in the case of ex-POWs in 1945-6 has undoubtedly helped to prevent much demoralisation in the community: an extension of the CRUs to all members of all services would undoubtedly have prevented much more.

HOW SHALL WE DEAL WITH THE "DISRUPTIVES"?

The technical problems of handling unresolved aggression in children, adolescents and adults are being much considered to-day by medical psychologists. At the moment this chapter is being revised, an International Conference on Child Psychiatry is devoting all its sessions to this topic alone.

Yet once the need for such handling is recognised, the actual techniques are not in themselves difficult. Most Child Guidance clinics, more especially those experienced in play therapy, are well able—with some help from parents, school etc.—to cope with aggressive manifestations in children. Eventually their influence should eliminate many of the factors that create "disruptive" adults.

In the adolescent, the problem has already become much more difficult since it has invaded a larger, less controllable social environment. Constructive group activities are the greatest single help: reinforced where necessary by special individual therapy and by control and modification of the social environment. On the higher levels of leadership, the disruptives and the aggressive psychopaths—especially in their subtler manifestations—should especially be watched for: and where found by screening, given special placement, therapy if required or—in the last issue—controlled and supervised. It may be more comfortable for the disruptive that his aggression be turned outwards but it is worse for society: if turned in, it can disrupt only his own personality, if turned out it will add to the disruptive forces of society: unless and until it can be constructively canalised.

The regime of Hitler, Goebbels and Goering is a large-scale object-lesson of the danger of allowing aggressive psychopaths to high office: and of *the plausible appeal of their extroverted aggression* and mis-leadership to some politicians and men of action—especially the unsubtle, the unstable and the psychologically obtuse—and *to the unresolved aggression in ordinary people when appealed to as mobs*. It points incidentally to the need to distinguish between success in adjustment and social value. A Hitler is relatively well adjusted for a time though his social effect is negative. The adjusted but disruptive psychopath may at first sight present to many a more plausible figure than the self-driving creative neurotic: but the latter, though poorly adjusted, is making a positive contribution, and most of the world's intellectual and aesthetic pioneering is done by his type. But once screened, it is important that the "disruptives" be used: certainly not rejected. Unresolved aggression is, after all, energy balked of its creative and cooperative outlet: here is the clue to its use.

No expense would have been too great to pay for a psychotherapy or a sociotherapy that might have modified or prevented or perhaps even cured a Hitler. No community can afford not to spare whatever trouble or expense is required to curb and redirect the destructive power of "disruptives" haunted by the compulsion to throw spanners into cooperative living; for their potentialities for destruction are so very considerable.

In using "disruptives" it is important that they should be

given special attention and help, special placement and observation and follow-up, special therapy or training where they require it; and, in the last issue, special control and supervision where nothing else avails. The likelihood is that the greater percentage of them—who are mildly "bloody-minded"—will respond to kindly and careful placement, to an invitation to more effective participation and to a planned progression in shared responsibility.

IN WHOSE INTERESTS SHALL SELECTION OPERATE?

"Vocational guidance" is finding a job for the individual, "vocational selection" is finding an individual for the job. One acts on behalf of the individual or employee, the other on behalf of the group or employer: in America they would be termed "client-centred" and "community-centred".

It seems important that no opposition or dissociation of interest between one and the other should be implied. In selecting for large public services and in educational schemes, it should not be difficult to consider both interests: provided the principle be accepted that both *should* be considered. In smaller private organisations, the need for a safeguarding machinery will arise.

Alternative terms—to avoid the connotation of either "guidance" or "selection"—may have to be thought out. Tentatively one suggests "guidance *and* allocation" or "vocational examination" or "occupational screening".

This conjunction of interests suggests:—

a that, where possible, men be screened for all levels (as in the Army where it is done in two phases) so that there may be little or no need for absolute rejections:

b that those screened be given individual guidance in the light of the information gained.

NO MAN'S FATE MUST DEPEND ON ONE SELECTION SCREENING

It is important that no one should feel that a selection procedure has sealed his fate for all time. If selection is not able to open—*and keep on opening*—gates to opportunity, its existence is not fully justified. As the number of those placed in jobs above their true level is relatively few in any community to-day; and the number of those placed in jobs below their potential level relatively many, it should not be difficult for selection to offer an avenue of reasonable hope.

As a democratic filter to help the individual to find fruitful and satisfying roles in the community, any comprehensive scheme of selection needs multiple screens at various periods to allow for (a) the percentage of error inherent in any predictive procedure, (b) the unpredictable elements in maturation and its tempo, (c) the variable factors in training, (d) the influence of therapeutic procedures and other auxiliaries to training, (e) changes due to health, accident, act of Providence, etc.

When these screens should be used, is a matter for further investigation. Some of the possibilities are:—

a In early school life—about 11—as a rough check and guide to further educational needs: not to be interpreted rigidly or definitively on any one test without reference to health, emotional and social attitudes and the whole picture and background.

b Some time before leaving school—possibly 15 to 16—to determine vocational trends and allow for appropriate preliminary education.

c On entering a vocation or profession.

d In certain fields, after a preliminary training, where allocation to leadership level is still possible for slow developers and others.

e At any period where change of health, maladjustment in the job, automatic eligibility for change of status or level by seniority, etc. demand a re-allocation.

If these screens are used for individual guidance as well as for allocation, their value will be considerably enhanced.

THE MEDICAL PSYCHOLOGIST AND SELECTION

To the medical psychologist, Selection is an important aspect of constructive social medicine: and, for "the complex 25%," an actual sociotherapy which should stabilise them. It is in helping Selection Boards to solve the problems of the latter that he can call attention to the interpersonal and intrapersonal frictions and conflicts that may unstabilise anybody.

Medical psychology has something to learn here as well as to give. WOSB paper screening with its Projection Battery could —if suitably modified—save many psychotherapeutic man-hours badly needed for other patients. The basic screening data—age, intelligence, education, socio-economic status etc—could be Hollerithed as in WOSB and thus made available for almost automatic analysis and routine research. All this would use the psychologist more effectively, bring him into the therapeutic team and "picture", and feed him with the experience he needs for participation of this kind.

It might be useful to attempt a short-term validation of therapists and the effects of their treatment as well as a long-term validation of procedures and even of "Schools": which should assist both. It should not be difficult to devise a useful 3- or 4-point rating of therapeutic effect (possibly in terms of relief of personal suffering, improvement in functional level on the job, improved group-cohesiveness and social relations).

The therapeutic team *as team* seems worthy of further encouragement and experimentation: which group therapy would facilitate. This would distribute the therapeutic burden, might simplify some aspects of the transference and counter-transference: and would provide the patient with a "micro-community" of patients and therapists in which to make his first faltering attempts to get on better terms with his community.

SELECTION SHOULD OPERATE AS A DEMOCRATIC FILTER

In so far as a scheme of selection helps all to play their part in collective leadership and collective achievement, it will make a reality of the incentive "Every Man a Leader" and "all are called and all may be chosen": it will act as a truly democratic filter.

What it must not do—or seem to do—has already been mentioned. What it must do—and seem to do—is to help *all* in the community to their happiest and most useful level and field: to reinforce that help with individual guidance: and to allow amply for every possibility of error, every change in circumstance, every tempo of development, every birth of new ambition.

However efficient a selection procedure, it can only select those who *should* become leaders: it cannot hope to prophesy those who *will*, nor need it be expected to. In the first few lines of this book, we suggested that leadership—like intelligence and every other human function—is inherited only as a potentiality: it must be discovered, cherished, trained and given scope. The onus of discovering that potentiality rests on selection: that of training it skilfully and providing the opportunities that will extend it fully must rest on the community.

CHAPTER XXIII

A NOTE OF COORDINATION

The object of this chapter is not to summarise the book but to coordinate certain topics discussed throughout it. Chapter numbers are in brackets.

LEVEL OF GROUP EFFECTIVENESS OR LEADERSHIP

Leadership is equated with group-effectiveness and its 3 aspects: functional level, group-cohesiveness and stability.

Functional Level

Four aspects are considered:—

a A means of indicating *potential* functional capacity by an index compounded of intelligence level and educational standard, both on officer, professional or managerial level (8 and 14) and on NCO, technician or foreman level (21).

b Functional roles or the various phases of functional capacities in action, i.e. planning, organising, practical execution, etc. (5 and 12). Further aspects of functional roles are considered in relation to group-management principles (13): see also page 269.

c The effect on stability of the inter-relationship between (1) *potential* functional level, (2) *actual* functional level, (3) the functional level *aspired* to, (4) the level *required* by the task or job, (5) the objectivity of the candidate's *self-estimated* level (12 and 14).

d An approach to the study of attitudes and their effect on functional level in special fields (pages 118, 253).

Group-cohesiveness

Three aspects are considered:—

a Social roles required in high degree of those who function on leadership level, i.e. empathy, encouragement, firmness, tact, etc (13 and 14).

b Two parallel typologies of personality for use in ratings of group performance and in psychological profiles:—

1 the first, a sociodynamic one, in terms of the attitude to the group i.e. cohesive, disruptive, dependent or isolate (5 and 10).

2 the second in terms of the psychodynamic make-up determining that attitude to the group, i.e. MATCOP IMAG and IMDEP (14).

c Positive behavioral signs of superior adjustment to the group i.e. warmth, spontaneity, objectivity, cooperativeness and commensurate effectiveness (14).

Stability

The following aspects of stability are considered:—

a The nature of neurosis and health in relation to participation and leadership in the group (3, 4, 5, 22).

b The principal contributory factors to instability (5, 14).

c The evaluation of these factors from:—

1 written "background" and "projective" material (8):

2 behaviour in response to the Stress Group Task and its impasses (5 and 10):

3 the psychiatric interview (14).

d Notes on therapy and rehabilitation (3, 22, page 186).

ITS MEASUREMENT

A measurable index to potential *Functional Level* in terms of intelligence and education is mentioned above (8, 14, 21).

The best approach to the evaluation of *Group-cohesiveness* is through techniques of "projecting" characteristic emotional and social attitudes in writing, speech, action and the expression of opinions and choices.

Written projection techniques are discussed as the "third screening element" in (8). Spoken projective techniques are considered in relation to the Undirected Group Discussion (9), the second phase of the Planning Project (12), the Human Problems Session (13) and the "projective" interview (14). All of these may reveal the presence or otherwise of the positive behavioral signs of superior adjustment already mentioned (14). The projection of social and emotional attitudes in action is a prime purpose of the Stress Group Task (5, 9, 10, 12, 16): though it throws light also on functional behaviour and level. The projection and measurement of attitudes—both of individuals and the groups that contain them—from their expression in choices and opinions is attempted in the Sociometric or Judgement Test (17).

The evaluation of *Stability* is a medical matter (14).

Three scales for rating Group-effectiveness as a whole are listed, compared (end of 8) and discussed (10, 18).

MEASURING THE RELIABILITY OF ITS MEASUREMENT

Validation is measurement of the reliability of measurements. It is discussed as such (20) and as an aid to training selectors (18).

APPLICATIONS OF FIELD OR GESTALT THEORY

To Group Inter-relationships

The inter-relationships between members of a working group are discussed (2, 3, 4, 5, 9, 10, 12, 13, 14, etc.). These relationships are primarily functional, i.e. in direct relation to the task or LOTS (5, 12, 13): and secondarily social, i.e. to evoke, direct and implement functional capacities.

To Testing Procedure

The planning of test procedure is discussed under the heading "The Psychology of 3-phase Testing" (6). The differentiation of the testing pattern into its inter-related components is accompanied by a parallel differentiation of the observer team into its specialist functions.

To Screening Procedure

The type of collective thinking required and its effective co-ordination in screening procedures is indicated in respect of the Query Conference (11), the Interim Grading (15) and the Final Board (18). A new Psychological Profile for testing and screening purposes is suggested (18). The theory of screening is discussed in these 3 chapters and epitomised at the beginning of Chapter XIV. Both data and observer team are differentiated into their parts and related to each other. It is interesting that the WOSB observer team could exemplify in the handling of its own collective task, the approach which it looked for in those it judged.

To a Formulation of Group-management Principles

It is suggested (13) that if the LOTS (group-task) is differentiated into its component functions and these related to the capacities of the group, with the allocation of function goes its appropriate authority and responsibility. The dynamic and interdependent nature of imperatives, orders, commands, directives, etc. is considered.   Control is regarded as the limiting effect of each function on every other function, and between whole and part functions: Power as the potential energy deriving from the coordination of individual functional abilities in the group in relation to a task.

RECORDING TECHNIQUES

Recording Tests:—
    Undirected Group Discussion (9, 10).
    Progressive Group Task (9, 10).
    Apparatus Session (12).
    Judgement Test—as a test (17).

Recording Screening Procedures:—
    Query Conference (11).
    Interim Grading Slip (15).
    Judgement Test—as a screen (17).
    Final Board (18).

Reportage:—
    of the Group (10).
    of the Candidate (14, 18).

BIBLIOGRAPHIC NOTE

The prime source of material is one's experience of WOSB: one is indebted also to technical memoranda issued by its Research and Training Centre.

Application of the field approach to dynamic psychology has been adumbrated by KURT LEWIN in books and papers, of which the following constitute a useful introduction:—

1 A Dynamic Theory of Personality. New York, 1935.
2 Principles of Topological Psychology. New York, 1936.
3 The Conceptual Representation and Measurement of Psychological Forces. Duke Univ. Press, 1938.

A simpler exposition of the Lewinian approach is contained in the first part of:

4 BROWN, J. F. Psychology and the Social Order, 1936.

The Judgement Test derives from J. L. MORENO: and the Human Problems Session has elements in common with his "psychodrama" and "sociodrama". A stimulating conspectus of his views is given in:—

5 Who Shall Survive? 1934.

A useful analysis of the choice process in the sociometric test is given by H. H. JENNINGS—a co-worker of Moreno—in:

6 Leadership and Isolation, 1943. New York: Longmans.

Discussed in the text are the following:—

7 FRENCH, J. R. P. The Disruption and Cohesion of Groups. Journ. Abnorm. Soc. Psychology, Vol. 36, p. 362–377; July, 1941. This discusses an experimental study of the emotional behaviour of two types of groups—organised and unorganised (i.e. leaderless groups)—when presented with situations producing frustration. The frustration was produced by requiring the groups to solve insoluble problems which they were led to believe were soluble. Various types of disruptive and cohesive behaviour are described.

8 T. E. COFFIN. A Three-Component Theory of Leadership. Journ. Abn. Soc. Psych. Vol. 39, p. 63–83; June 1944.

9 Dynamic Administration: The Collected Papers of MARY PARKER FOLLETT. Edited by L. Urwick and H. C. Metcalf. 1941, London.

10 SIDNEY HOOK. The Hero in History. 1943.

Of relevant interest are:

11 L. URWICK. The Elements of Administration. 1943, London.

12 SIR OLIVER FRANKS. Central Planning and Control in War and Peace. 1947, London.

13 R. G. COLLINGWOOD. An Autobiography. Chapter v. 1939.

14 SIR GEORGE SCHUSTER. Human Relations in Industry. Brit. Med. Journ., Sept. 11, 1948.

APPENDIX A

A SPECTRUM RATING OF OFFICER PERSONALITY

Superior

RED — Superior—all round: in most fields or officer roles.

ORANGE — Superior—in a limited field, i.e. technical or special arm.

Acceptable

YELLOW — Good average—good in most officer roles.

GREEN — Low average: fair at most things—but with some limitations: or—average in a limited field.

BLUE — Borderline—might do if with compensatory features i.e. unusually good contact, firm character, special experience, physical drive, etc.

Unsuitable

INDIGO A — *Limited personality.*
1 Weak—"dim", "wet": so inhibited socially or emotionally as to be unable to realise his potentialities.
2 NCO—of low potential level and limited range of outlook.
3 In a rut—by age, stereotyped attitude or type of experience.
4 OIR too low for officer level i.e. OIR 1 or 2.
5 Gleam of hope: *might* come up again under his own steam: not as likely to do so as NY.
6 Strong personality and drive but egocentric, antisocial, difficult and generally group-disruptive.

INDIGO B   *Nervous personality.*
1 Psychosomatic or hysteric.
2 Anxious or obsessional.
3 Labile—mood swings.
4 "Schizoid" or "Shut-in" type.

Unsuitable
(*continued*)

VIOLET   *Manifestly psychiatric.*
1 Severe anxiety or obsessional.
2 Severe labile.
3 Schizoid, paranoid, or psychopathic personality.

N.B.—If the candidate is immature, but likely to develop, the grading should be preceded by NY (not yet) i.e. NY/Y means that when he does mature, he will function on Yellow level.

APPENDIX B

TEST OF OBJECTIVE JUDGEMENT [Page 1]

Course No...... Cand. No......

1 *An officer must be capable of objective judgement:* he must be able to distinguish between his liking for a man and his estimate of that man's ability to do a job: he must be able to drink with a man one evening and decide on his capacity for a vital job next morning. Only in this way can he hope to pick the right man for the right job.

2 *The object of this test is to estimate your capacity for the objective judgement of men.* Your PSO has now made up his mind about all of you; his only way of estimating *your* judgement is by comparing it with his.

3 In Table I, *rank the other members of your group in the order in which you would appreciate their friendship* and would like to work with them as pals or colleagues.

As FRIEND		As OFFICER or as LEADER		Reasons for FIRST choice as LEADER
1		1		
2		2		
3		3		
4		4		
5		5		Reasons for LAST choice as LEADER
6		6		
7		7		
8		8		
9		9		

275

4 In Table II, *rank them in the order in which you would respect their leadership and would like to work under them.*

5 As an even more delicate test of the objectivity of your judgement, after you have ranked as in 3 and 4, go over each ranking again and divide it with 3 brackets into 3 groups (a), (b) and (c). (a) are those you would particularly like as friend or leader: (b) are those you could work with but would not particularly choose: (c) are those—if any—with whom you would not particularly care to work or might find difficult.

6 The other questions explain themselves.

[Page 2]

A Write—as if on a postcard to your parents or pal—an account of how you got on at WOSB: comment on your own performance and mention any factors, adverse or otherwise, that may have influenced it.

B Which features of WOSB (tests, paper-work, interviews, etc.) seem to you most useful in selecting officers and why? Which seem least useful and why? Have you any suggestions to make?

C Have you any frank comments or criticisms to make of WOSB generally or of conditions during your stay here?

APPENDIX C THE PROFILE PROFORMA

BACKGROUND SUMMARY.

No... Rank..

Name... Age................. Med. Cat................. OIR............................

Regt/Corps... Choice of Arm..

1. MILITARY SERVICE (inc. Pre-Service)

2. EDUCATION

3. OCCUPATION

4. SOCIAL PARTICIPATION

5. SPORTS

6. HOBBIES

7. FAMILY BACKGROUND

[Page 2]

PROFILE REPORT ON CANDIDATE FOR O.C.T.U.

Name_____ No._____ W.O.S.B. Course No._____ Cand. No._____

SUITABILITY FOR O.C.T.U.	G	S	B	W	V.W.	REMARKS
1. Leadership experience						
2. Unit Report						
3. O.I.R.						
4. Educational suitability						
5. Planning ability						
6. Practical ability						
7. Athletic ability						
8. Level of aims						
9. Effectiveness in pursuit of aims						
10. Military Compatibility						
11. Sense of Responsibility						
12. Social Interest						
13. Quality of personal relations						
14. Range of personal relations						
15. Dominance						
16. Liveliness						
17. Stability of Health						

SUMMING UP.

_____

_____

_____

_____

_____

_____

_____

_____

_____

_____

MEMBER'S PRE-BOARD RECOMMENDATION	MEMBERS' FINAL GRADING	BOARD FINAL DISPOSAL
Suitable	Team Leader ...	GRADE ... ...
Doubtful ...	M.T.O.	ARM ... ...
Unsuitable ...	Psych.	

President.
Team Leader.
Psych.
M.T.O.

Date_____   Signed_____

APPENDIX D

THE INTERIM GRADING SLIP

Interim Grading Slip

GROUP A

CAND. NO.	PRES.	MTO.	PSYCH.
1			
2			
3			
4			
5			
6			
7			
8			
9			

Interim Grading Slip

GROUP B

CAND. NO.	PRES.	MTO.	PSYCH.
21	C	D	C
22	F	F	
23	F	DD	D ✳
24	C	C	—
25	B	C	—
26	D	F.	— ✳
27	C	D	—
28	NY	DD	D ✳
29			

Interim Grading Slip

GROUP C

CAND. NO.	PRES.	MTO.	PSYCH.
31			
32			
33			
34			
35			
36			
37			
38			
39			

This example illustrates the use of the slip. Gradings are as defined on page 216. Where there is substantial agreement of opinion, a line is drawn through the gradings. Those about whom there is serious difference of opinion are starred for special observation in the Final Exercise. If, after this, there is still disagreement and the candidate has not been interviewed psychologically, he now is interviewed for a third opinion.

APPENDIX E

A SHORT INTERESTS QUESTIONNAIRE

[Page 1]

Name................Course No......Cand. No......

Write a 5 minute essay on your favourite games, sports, hobbies and interests: indoor and outdoor: in the order in which they interest you.

[Page 2]

(A blank page for special "projective" questions to be given orally by the Serjeant-Tester).

A SHORT INTERESTS QUESTIONNAIRE

1 What influenced you in the choice of your civilian career? Were you satisfied with it? If not, why?

2 What career would you have chosen had you been quite free to choose? What prevented you from doing so?

3 What occupation do you hope to follow on leaving the Army? What do you hope to be doing in 20 years' time?

4 What events in your life do you regard as (a) "High Spots" (b) "Low Spots" (c) "Critical or worrying events"? Give examples.

   a

   b

   c

5 What persons or events have influenced your life (a) for the better, (b) for the worse?

   a

   b

6 Describe any person in history, fiction or fact (a) whom you look up to as a type to be admired, (b) whom you dislike intensely.

   a

   b

A SHORT INTERESTS QUESTIONNAIRE

7 What motto, phrase or proverb most nearly sums up your attitude to life?

8 What is the object of your life?

9 How do you think your Army experience will affect your attitude to your civilian job?

10 When you leave the Army, what features of Army life—if any—are you most likely to miss.

11 What is there about the officer's job,

    a That appeals to you most

    b That you feel most confident about

    c That you feel least confident about

12 What advice would you give to a younger brother just about to enter the Army?

13 One or two of the above questions may be unimportant in your case. Give one question which you think would be more suitable.

NAME INDEX

Bion, W. R., 2, 26
Brown, J. F., 6, 271

Chiang Yee, 71
Coffin, T. E., 31, 271
Collingwood, R. G., 272

Dostoevsky, 168

Follett, M. P., 139, 259, 271
Franks, Sir Oliver, 272
French, J. R. P., 26, 271
Freud, 6

Goethe, 71, 172
Goncharov, 177

Hamlet, 169
Hook, S., 256, 272

Jennings, H. H., 208, 271

Lady Macbeth, 169
Lewin, K., 6, 271

Metcalf, H. C., 139, 271
Millar, W. M., 72
Moreno, L., 125, 147, 202, 208, 271
Myers, L. H., 174

Reeve, G., 3, Chapter 20
Rickman, J., 15, 156
Robbins, C. W., 124
Rodger, F., 2, 16

Schilder, P., 15, 16, 27
Schiller, 71
Schuster, Sir George, 272
Shakespeare, 172
Spranger, 64
Sutherland, J. D., 2, 3, 26

Trist, E., 2, 16, 26

Urwick, L., 139, 272

Wilson, A. T. M., 16
Wittkower, E., 2

SUBJECT INDEX

Acceptability, 204
Accident-proneness, 169
Ambivalence, 159
Apparatus Session, 118
Aptitudes, 8, 18, 32, 253
Atmosphere, selection versus training, 49
Attitudes
— in relation to aptitudes, 119, 252
— social and vocational, 252
Authority, 141, 181, 216, 269

Background Summary, 53
Basic Family Attitudes (BFA), 154, 158
Basic Interpersonal Attitudes (BIA), 61, 154, 158, 160
Basic Series, 41, chap 9
— compared with Command Situations, 112
— compared with Final Exercise, 98
Biography, 57, 175, 214
Briefing
— and the time incentive, 91
—" phantasy," 82, 90
— the Human Problems Session, 126
— the Judgement Test, 202
— the Progressive Group Task, 82
— the Undirected Group Discussion, 76
Bulletin Board, 198

Candidates
— " abreacting " ones attitude to, 77, 86
— differential diagnosis of shy types, 105
— immature or NY (Not Yet) types, 95, Appendix A
— miscellaneous types in the Stress Group Task, 94
Causality, 20, 46
Civil Rehabilitation Units (CRU), 16, 262
Collective
— effort, 231

Collective—
— leadership, 142, chap 22
— thinking, 211
Command Situations (CS), 110
Commensurate Effectiveness, 165, 176, 178, 225
Conflict and the group's problems, 140
Control, 141, 270
Conversation, 'points to observe in, 68
Cooperativeness, 165, 175, 178, 232
CO's Report, 60
Counter-transference, 162

" Dominant Values," 64
Drive, 183, 226

Educational Standard (ES) qv Level Required, 57
Empathy, 132, 137
Encouragement, capacity for, 132, 137
Ex-POWs qv CRU, 18
Expressive movements, 169

Field, three uses of the word, 22
Final Board (FB), 44, chap 18, Appendix C
Final Exercise (FE), 43, 200
— relaxes group and team, 201
Firmness, capacity for, 133, 138
Function defined, 132, 141
— distinguished from role, 141

GABI rank-rating, 72, 80, 84, 97, 102, 198, 213, 214, 219, 223–4
Group-cohesiveness, 11, 29, 30, 36, 92, 104, 109, 125, 149, 154, 166, 181, 185, 202, 225, 267.
Group-cohesive personality, 30, 36, 92, 140, 202
Group-dependent personality, 31, 37, 94
Group-disruptive personality, 31, 37, 93, 140, 262

Group Dossier, 214
Group-effectiveness, 10, 13, 23, 28, 72, 74, 257.
"Group equation," 168, 206
Group-management, 139–43, 147
— defined, 138
Groups, superior and poor, 179

Handwriting as a pointer, 71, 168–9
Health Record qv Stability, psychosomatic pointers to, 59
Human Problems Session (HPS), 29, 43, 116, chap 13, 168, 170, 174

IMAG, 159–65, 177, 179–80, 208, 268
IMDEP, 159, 161–3, 177–9, 208, 268
Impasse, 33
Imperatives to the group, 141
Incentives, 138–9, chap 22
Individuality and the group, 25
Indolence Test, 35
Intelligence Level, 54
Interests
— Questionnaire (IQ) 63, appendix E
— Session, 115
Interim Grading and Slip, 43, chap 15, appendix D
Interviews
— group, 115, 129
— linked, 122
— projective, chap 14
— psychiatric
— — candidate's anxiety about, 108
— — graded priorities for, 106–7, 150
— — of superior candidates, 107, 164
— — referrals for, 150, 201
— technical, 121
— therapeutic, 15
Intra-Group Race, 41, 81
Intuition, 79, 88, 98, 255
Isolate, 31, 94

Judo, 155, 157, 170–1,
Judgement Test, 44, 168, 172, chap 17, 269, appendix B
Law of the Total Situation (LOTS), 110, 137, 139–43
"Leader" not a useful word in Selection, 27

Leadership
— a collective function, 109, 257
— and attitude to conflict, 142
— and dominance, 28, 138, 222–3
— and followership, 19, 112, 160
— and "Führer-prinzip," 259
— and the healthy personality, 24, 257
— a series, not a dichotomy, 20
— defined, 19, 25
— g factors in, 22, 251
— "institutional," 142
— its evolution, 255
— lower limits of, qv Level of Functioning Required, 21
— roles, training in, 147
— s factors in, 23, 251
Leisure, use of, 260
Level of functioning, 10, 20, 29, 149–54, 188, 225, 267–8
— and stability, qv
— and the Level Cluster, 225
— and the Stress Group Task, 91
— Actual, 151–2
— Aspired, 151–3
— as sampled in the Interview, 153
— Opted, 151
— optimum, 38
— Potential, 151
— Required, 151
— — on foreman, NCO or technician level, 218, 254, 267
— — on officer, manager or professional level, 57, 152, 267
— queries about, 103
— Self-estimated, 151, 153
— varies with the field, 22, 30
Losing ones temper constructively, 138

Man-management
— defined, 138
— techniques of, 136–9, 147
MATCOP, 159, 162, 167, 177, 180, 208, 268
Medical psychologist
— and selection generally, 14, 229, 232, 265

Medical psychologist
— double function in the community, 13
— objectivity a sine qua non, 174
— redressing the balance of his experience, 164-5, 230
— talk to candidates, 50
Morale, 181, 185
— versus predisposition, 182
Motivation in relation to the job, 134
Muga, 171

Neurosis
— causes, in terms of the group, 11
— defined, in terms of the group, 25
— group therapy in, 14
— therapy by a team, 266
— treatment of, in terms of the group, 11, 13-16, 186
— use of WOSB techniques in treatment, 265

Objectivity of social thinking, 165, 172, 178
— and commonsense, 173
— and humour, 173
Oblomovism, 177
Observer teams
— role in the Stress Group Task, 85
— types of, 179
Obstacles
— " double-entry," 83, 200
— " narrow-entry," 83
— " shake-down," 200
— " wide-area," 83, 200
— " wide-entry," 82, 200
Officer Intelligence Rating (OIR) qv Level Required, 56
Orders, 141-2
Organising, 31-2, 140

Past Record, 57-60, 214, 220, 225
Pen-picture, 194, 215
Personality
— " engineering," 24, 118
— in terms of field psychology, 7
— Pointers, 53, 72
— superior or mature, 163-179

Personnel Selection Officer (PSO)
— age, 89
— Battery, 110-120
— general functions, 39
— intelligence, 88
— role in the Stress Group Task, 86-91
Persuasion, 31-2
Planning, 31, 140
— Project (PP), 29, 116
Practical execution, 32
Progressive Group Task (PGT), 28, 41, 80
Projection
— Battery, 61-71, 170, 265
— defined, 61
— interpretation of 70
— techniques, 61-70, 268
— — as the germinating point of leadership testing, 60, 90, 144, 202
— questions, 64, 188
Psychodynamics, 158, 268
— and sociodynamics, 158
— of competitiveness, 258-9
Psychological
— department, 39, chap 19
— jargon, 197
— profile, 220
— — a suggested new, 224
Psychology
— and sociology, 5
— Associationist, 45
— " field " or Gestalt, 6, 45, 210, 224, 269
— of the 3-phase procedure, 45
— present trend in, 5
Pulheems, 115

Query Conference, 42, chap 11, 109
— — proforma for, 102

Rating Techniques
— Final Board, 216
— Group-effectiveness qv GABI rank-rating and Spectrum Rating, 72
— social maturity qv
— stability, qv

Recording individual and group performance, 270
Rehabilitation qv CRU, 16, 186
Relating people to the LOTS (i.e. Law of the Total Situation)
— emotionally (" bringing others into the picture "), 31, 110, 133, 138, 225, 269
— functionally, 31, 110, 133, 138, 225, 169
Responsibility, 141, 181, 216, 269
— sense of, 221
Roles
— and functions distinguished, 132
— definition, 132
— distinguish enacted and projected roles, 128
—social, 32, 104, 132, 136–9

Sanity, positive signs of, 163–179, 268
Schools, boarding versus day, 59, 175
Screening
— one screen not enough, 265
— paper, 40, chap 8
— theory of, 42, 81, 149, 201, 204, 210–12
— three screening elements, 52, 54, 57, 60
Selection
— and constructive social medicine, 14, 17, 104, 186, 265
— and skimming the cream, 261
— and the weak links, 261
— a psychological job, 232
— as a democratic filter, 260, 266
— cannot function efficiently without psychological supervision, 232
— in boards without psychological supervision, 233
— in the Army
— — in Army Selection Centres (ASC), 18
— — in Primary Training Centres (PTC), 8, 18
— — on two levels, 8
— of women on leadership level, 255
— on foreman, NCO and technician level qv Level

Selection
— on officer, managerial and professional level qv Level
— requires medical help, 232
Selective Obstacles (SO), 113
Selectors
— age, 48, 89
— intelligence, 88
— temptation to " power-drunkenness," 89, 180
— Who will select the Selectors? 88
Self-description, 66, 173
Self-estimate qv Self-description, 208
Social maturity, 178
Sociatry and sociotherapy distinguished, 13
Sociodynamics, 158, 268
Sociometric approach, chap 17
Spectrum Rating, 72, 105, 218, appendix A
Spontaneity of expressive behaviour, 165, 168, 178, 225
— differential diagnosis of, 170
Stability, 11, 13, 33, 95, 181, 223, 226, 268
— and drive, 183, 226
— and group-cohesiveness, 11, 36, 92, 226
— and level, 181, 185, 226
— and morale, 181, 185, 226
— and the Stress Group Task, 95
— Cluster, 226
— global rating of, 185, 226
— in relation to the task, 37
— optimum, 38
— psychosomatic pointers to, 60, 104, 184
— queries about, 104
Stakhanovism, 259
Statistical analysis qv Validation, 71, 159, 185, 199, 217–8
Statisticians, *ad hoc* and *post hoc*, 230
Stress Group task qv Undirected Group Discussion, Progressive Group Task, Planning Project, Final Exercise etc., 8, chap 5, 175
— as " micro-community," 8, 26, 38
— " cramming " for, 96

Stress Group Task
— first experiments, 2, 26
— French's experiments, 26
— "sealing off," 86
— size of group, 26
— visitors observing, 77, 85, 126
Sumiye, 157, 171

Tact, capacity for, 133, 138
Tasks qv Obstacles
— "pseudo" and "real," 29
— planning, 82
Testing
— frustration in qv, impasse, 30
— results must be synergistically interpreted, 30, 71
— theory of, 149
"The bottom 10%," 262
"The complex 25%," 14, 17, 89, 104-5, 229, 265
Thematic Apperception Test (TAT), 68
"Therapeutic hint," 190
Typology of personality
— in psychodynamic terms, 158-163, 268
— in sociodynamic terms, 30, 36, 92, 140, 268

Undirected Group Discussion (UGD), 41, 74-80, 170
— as Stress Group Task, 28

Validation, chap 20
— defined, 234, 236, 269

Validation
— of therapy, 266
— short-term, as an aid to training selectors, 219
Vocational guidance v selection, 264

Warmth of feeling, 165, 166, 178
"Weighting" of global estimates, 120-2, 211
Word Association Test (WAT), 67
Worksheet for group-observation, 53
WOSB
— and the group approach, 7, 8, 10, 28
— constitution of, 39, 212
— first experiments, 2, 8, 26
— functions of
— — President, 39, 40, 45, 103, 211-2, 215-6
— — Deputy-president, 39, 103, 212-4
— — Senior PSO, 39, 212-4
— — Team-leader qv Deputy-president and Senior PSO
— — PSO qv
— — medical psychologist, 39-40, 50, 214-5, chaps 8, 14 and 19
— — psychologist, 40, 50, chaps 8, 14 and 19
— — Sergeant-Tester, 52-3, 107, 227
— three-phase procedure, 28, 40
"Wu-wei," 157, 171

Zen, 155, 157, 171